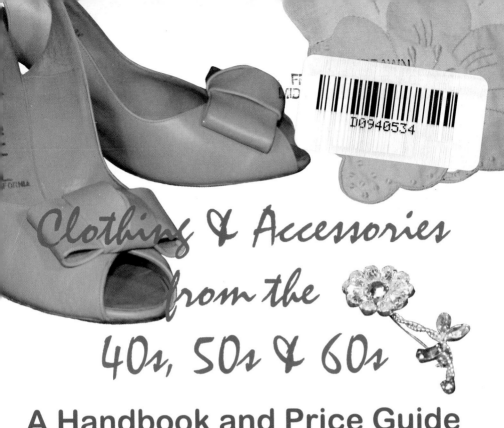

Clothing & Accessories from the 40s, 50s & 60s

A Handbook and Price Guide

Jan Lindenberger

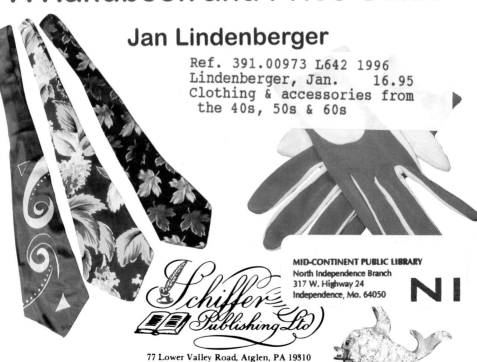

Schiffer Publishing Ltd

77 Lower Valley Road, Atglen, PA 19310

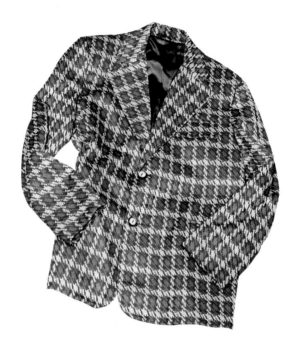

Printed in Hong Kong

ISBN: 0-7643-0023-7

Book Design by Audrey L. Whiteside

Library of Congress Cataloging-in-Publication Data

Lindenberger, Jan
    Clothing & accessories from the 40s, 50s & 60s: a handbook and price guide/Jan Lindenberger.
        p.   cm.
    ISBN 0-7643-0023-7 (paper)
    1. Costume--United States--History--20th century--Collectors and collecting--Catalogs. 2. Vintage clothing--United States--History--20th century--Collectors and collecting--Catalogs. 3. Dress accessories--United States--History--20th century--Collectors and collecting--Catalogs. I. Title.
GT615.L55   1996
391'.00973'09045--dc20   96-10490
                                          CIP

Published by Schiffer Publishing Ltd.
77 Lower Valley Road
Atglen, PA 19310
Please write for a free catalog.
This book may be purchased from the publisher.
Please include $2.95 for shipping.
Try your bookstore first.

We are interested in hearing from authors with book ideas on related subjects.

Contents

Introduction -- 4

Dresses -- 7

Blouses & Sweaters --- 31

Slips & Nightwear --- 39

Coats -- 46

Hats -- 50

Shoes -- 64

Purses --- 71

Scarves -- 87

Gloves --- 92

Sunglasses --- 96

Men's Clothing --- 98

Jewelry -- 102

Bibliography --- 128

Acknowledgments

A very special thank you to Joann Carson who owns "Mad Lidya's" in Colorado Springs, Colorado. Joann lent me her vast collection of clothing and accessories from both of her shops, "Discount Resales" and "Adobe Walls Antique Mall" in Colorado Springs, Colorado. Thanks also to Joyce and Jean Rosenthal from Lake Port, California for their kindness. Even though the hours were long, the great and informative conversations made it a joy to photograph their collection of vintage clothing and jewelry for this book. Last, but not least, I thank Cheryl Du Clusan, from Rancho Cordova, California. She was expecting her baby to be born anytime, but Cheryl took the time to lend me a hand dressing and undressing her mannequins. Her wonderful, varied collection of vintage hats, shoes and clothing from her shop in the Antique Plaza in Rancho Cordova, California was greatly appreciated.

Introduction

In the world of collecting clothing the word vintage has come to mean anything from the 1800s to the 1970s. Plastics from the 40s, 50s, and 60s are back and "in" again, as is the clothing from the same era. It's a well known fact that trends and fads will always make a come back.

The 1940s look was a lot of silk floral dresses, satin and rayon underslips, alligator shoes and purses. Beads accented clothing as did sequins. Coats and dresses were form fit and had a nice flowing style. File material hung well on suits and dresses and the clothing item usually had material buttons. Wide brim straw hats and feathers were stylish along with cotton gloves. Bakelite jewelry with the wide band bracelets were "vogue."

When the stylish fashions from the 1950s were all polyester pant suits we thought they were wonderful, but when they went out of style they went "out" of style! I never thought I would see the day when they would be back. Gone forever were elastic waists, bell bottom pants and loose boxed jackets. Never again would we see the preponderance of blues, browns, and dark colors, many of them checkered. I remember in the 50s and early 60s my daughter, Darlene, was not allowed to wear pants to school unless they were pant suits. And yes, they were polyester. It was not one of her favorite things to wear.

Imagine my surprise when, on a recent shopping trip in a fashionable store, those same designs and fabrics hung on many of the racks. Somehow it didn't do a thing for me, but several women and younger girls were trying them on and wearing them well. As for me, I'll wait!

In the 50s plastic jewelry, purses and belts were in, including plastic beads, bracelets and even rings. Sheer blouses, cummerbunds on dresses, high waistlines, and poodle skirts were popular. Toward the end of the 50s the colors were beginning to change from light to bright. Yellows, pinks and blues were fresh looking. Some new words on clothing labels were wash and wear, pre shrunk, polished cotton, washable, crisp, smart, and tailored. Those same words were used in the 60s.

The 50s and 60s crossed over in styles. Polyester was leaving and cotton shirtwaist dresses were holding their own. The dresses had gathered waists, wide square necklines and narrow material covered belts. Pleated skirts, boxed suits and jackets, pill box hats, cardigan sweaters, pegged capri slacks, and culotte skirts were in style. Gingham material was popular.

Plastic beads and rhinestone pins and necklaces also crossed over from the 50s into the 60s. Gloves were still being worn to accent outfits. Many short sets and skirt and blouses were color coordinated, along with color coordinated shoes. Buttons and bows were popular on oval toe shoes and pumps.

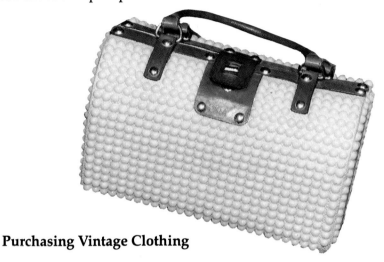

Purchasing Vintage Clothing

There are many important facts to remember when purchasing vintage clothing and accessories. Ask yourself if the item is all original? Have the buttons been changed? Has an angora or lace collar been added? Has the dress been double hemmed? Is it dry cleanable or washable? Maybe it's faded on the shoulders from being in a window display or on a hanger too long. Before buying an item check for tears, repairs, fading and wear.

Structure, style and design are important as well. If the item lasted this long and one takes special care of it while wearing and enjoying it, then it will remain a good vintage collectible. This also applies to jewelry, shoes, hats and other accessories.

The 40s, 50s, & 60s fashions are in style again in the 90s. The term "old clothing" is passe; the new term is "Vintage".

There are still some great "vintage buys" out there. Many antique shops have included clothing along with the general line of antiques and collectibles for sale. The flea markets have some great buys if you search them out. Auction houses are just now recognizing the value of vintage clothing and accessories, and these things are now appearing on their auction bills.

Prices may differ from area to area, and are affected by condition and availability. Shop prices differ from shows, flea markets and auctions.

Caring for Vintage Clothing

Here are some tips on caring for vintage clothing including cotton, linen and synthetic textiles. Most textiles will last for several years if cared for properly.

*Using acid free tissue and containers will prolong the life of the garment.

*Avoid stretching and putting stress on the garment by rolling or laying it flat.

*Keep container out of direct sunlight.

*Regular paper, cheap tissue, and cardboard will damage your textile.

*Wrap textiles in a clean washed sheet or acid free tissue.

*Don't leave garments in vinyl storage containers or plastic cleaner bags. You can find specialty storage bags at most cleaners.

*Avoid high humidity and temperature extreme areas to store your items. Air acids can weather or discolor items.

*Check your package regularly. Today's textiles will be tomorrow's treasures.

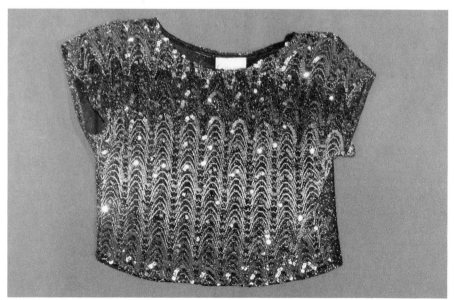

Dresses

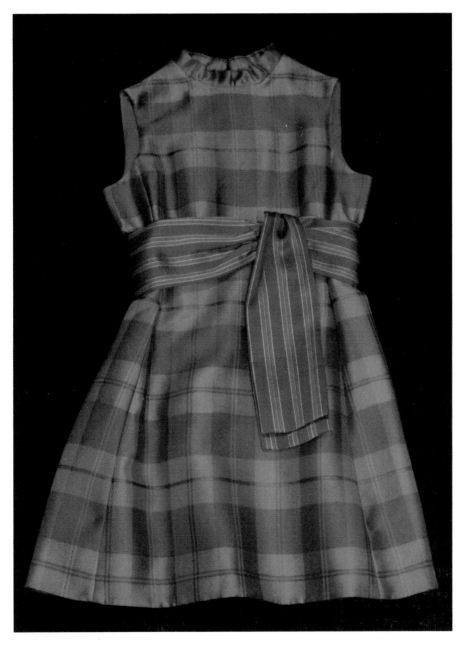

Sleeveless high waist dress. Wide tied front belt and zips up the back. 1960s. $20-30

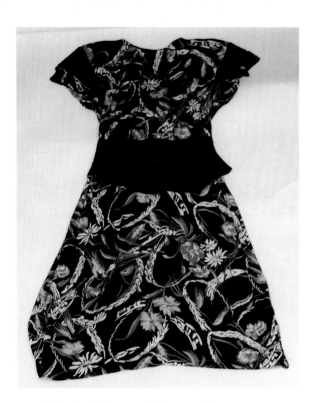

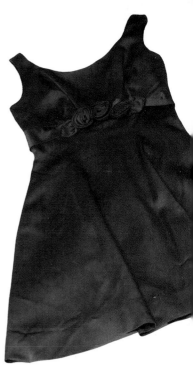

Silk floral drop waist dress with cap
sleeve. 1940s. $30-40

Green sheer floral cap sleeve dress.
Cotton flower near hem. 1960s. $40-50

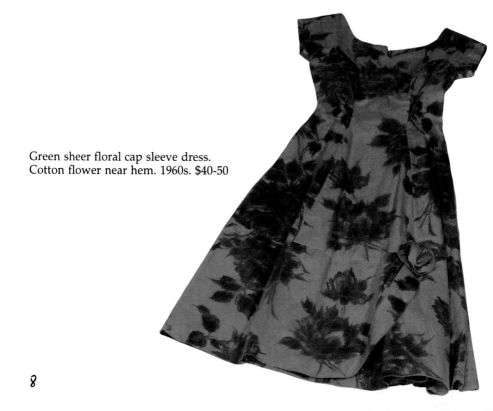

Velvet top of floral pleated dress with V neckline. 1950s. $20-30

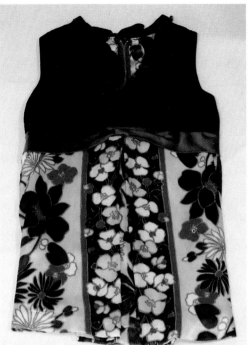

Blue satin A-line sleeveless dress. Satin bow at waistline. 1950s-60s. $30-40

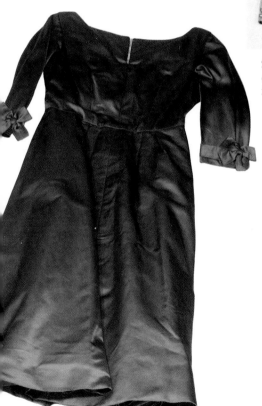

Strapless pink satin polka dot dress with stays in bust line and full skirt. 1950s. $20-30

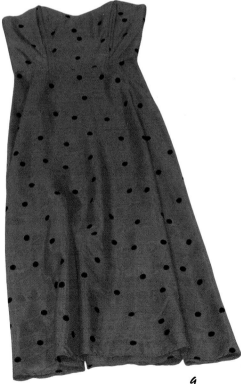

Satin low neck dress. Satin bows on sleeves. 1940s-50s. $20-30

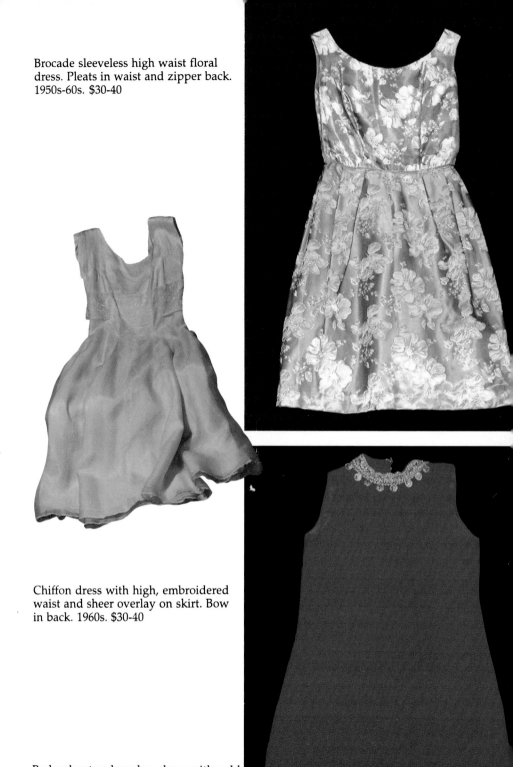

Brocade sleeveless high waist floral
dress. Pleats in waist and zipper back.
1950s-60s. $30-40

Chiffon dress with high, embroidered
waist and sheer overlay on skirt. Bow
in back. 1960s. $30-40

Red polyester sleeveless dress with gold
coin drop trim. Back bow and zipper.
1950s. $20-30

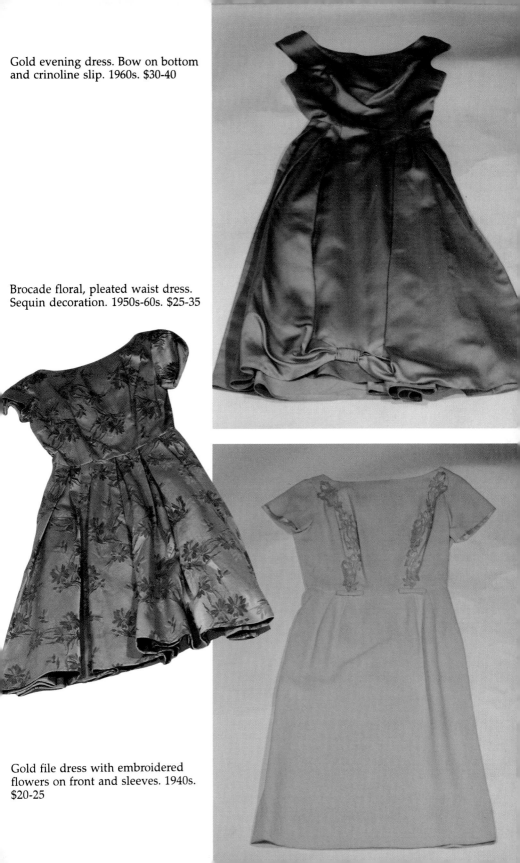

Gold evening dress. Bow on bottom and crinoline slip. 1960s. $30-40

Brocade floral, pleated waist dress. Sequin decoration. 1950s-60s. $25-35

Gold file dress with embroidered flowers on front and sleeves. 1940s. $20-25

Satin blend, A-line, sleeveless dress.
Material runs both ways. 1960s. $20-30

Wool dress with large round brass
buttons and long sleeves. 1940s. $45-55

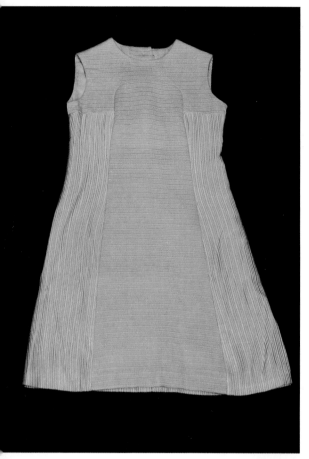

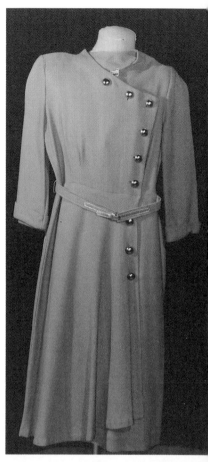

Orange chiffon long sleeve dress
trimmed down the front and on the
sleeves in gold piping. 1960s. $30-40

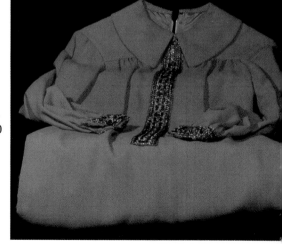

Pink and silver lace sheath dress. 1950s.
$35-45

Gold lace-over-silk-slip sleeveless
dress. 1960s. $20-30

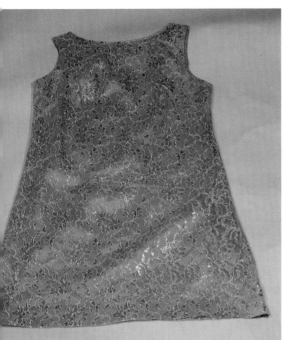

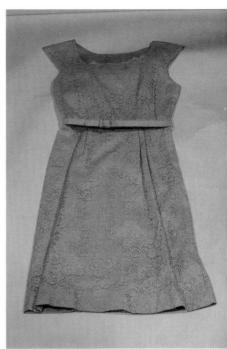

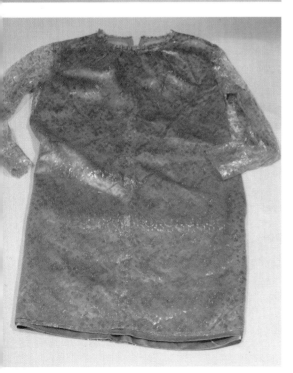

Orange and gold lace sheath
dress with high round collar
and satin underslip. 1960s. $25-
30.

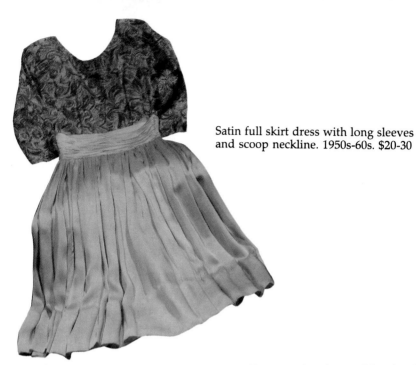

Satin full skirt dress with long sleeves and scoop neckline. 1950s-60s. $20-30

Brown satiny dress with velvet leaf design trim on neckline. 1940s. $30-40

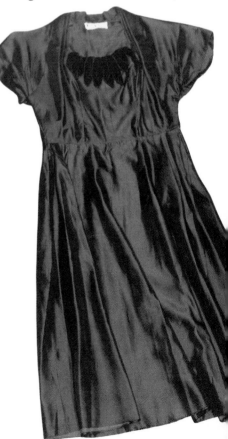

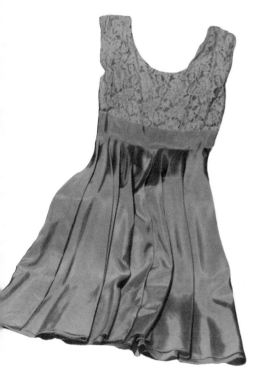

Taffeta sleeveless dress with lace top and bow in back. 1950s. $30-40

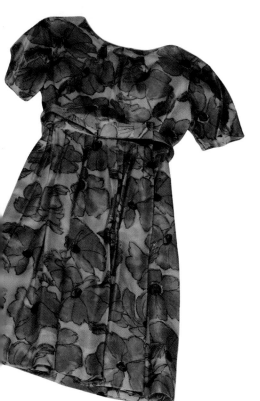

Long sleeve wool dress trimmed with beads and piping on shoulder. Beaded buttons. 1940s. $60-75

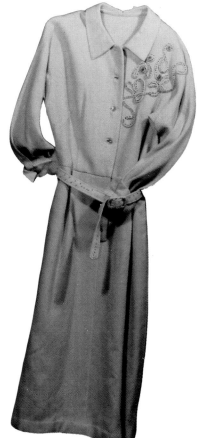

Green floral silk dress with self-belt, scoop neck and full skirt. 1960s. $30-40

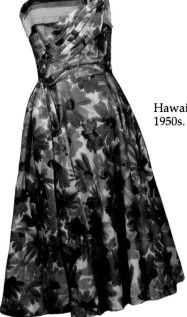

Hawaiian floral cotton strapless dress. 1950s. $30-40

Polka dot cotton button up dress. 1940s-50s. $20- 30

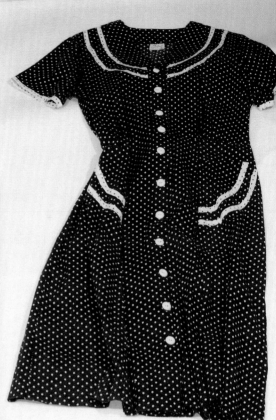

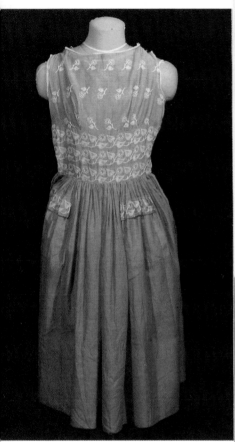

Orange cotton summer dress with embroidered pockets and bodice. 1960s. $15-20

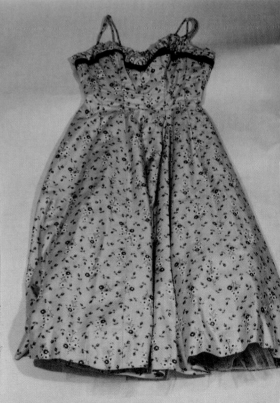

Spaghetti strap floral polished cotton sundress. Crinoline slip. Velvet trim and bow in back. 1960s. $30-40

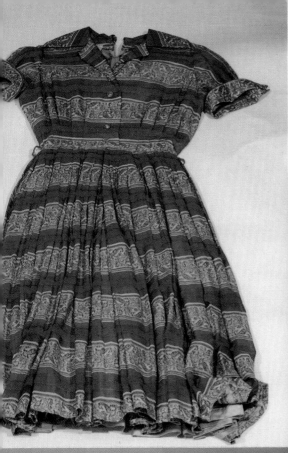

Shirtwaist short sleeve cotton dress with satin underslip. 1950s-60s. $30-40

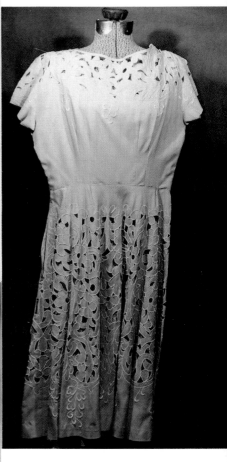

Embroidered cotton dress with cotton eyelet lace. 1940s-50s. $40-50

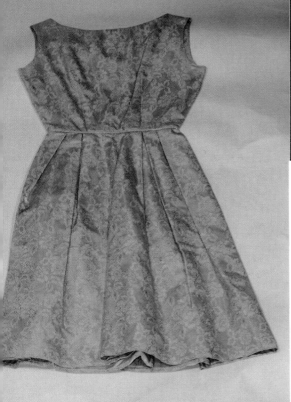

Green brocade sleeveless dress with full skirt. 1950s- 60s. $20-30

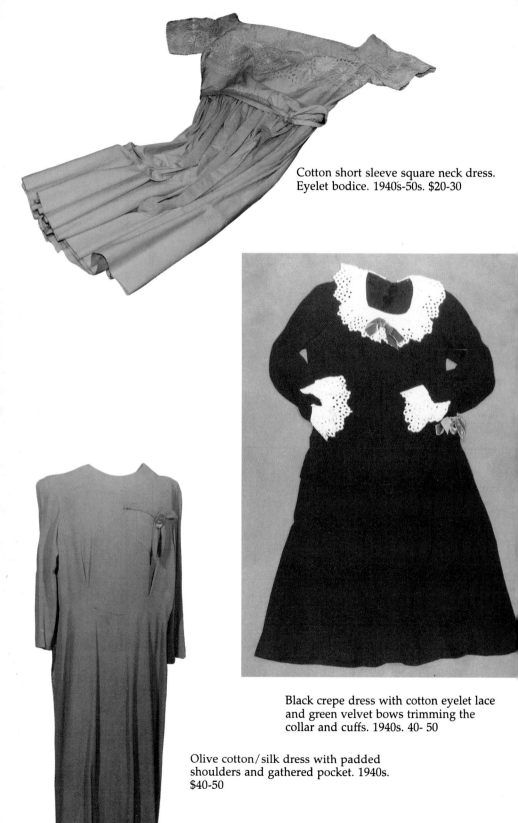

Cotton short sleeve square neck dress. Eyelet bodice. 1940s-50s. $20-30

Black crepe dress with cotton eyelet lace and green velvet bows trimming the collar and cuffs. 1940s. 40- 50

Olive cotton/silk dress with padded shoulders and gathered pocket. 1940s. $40-50

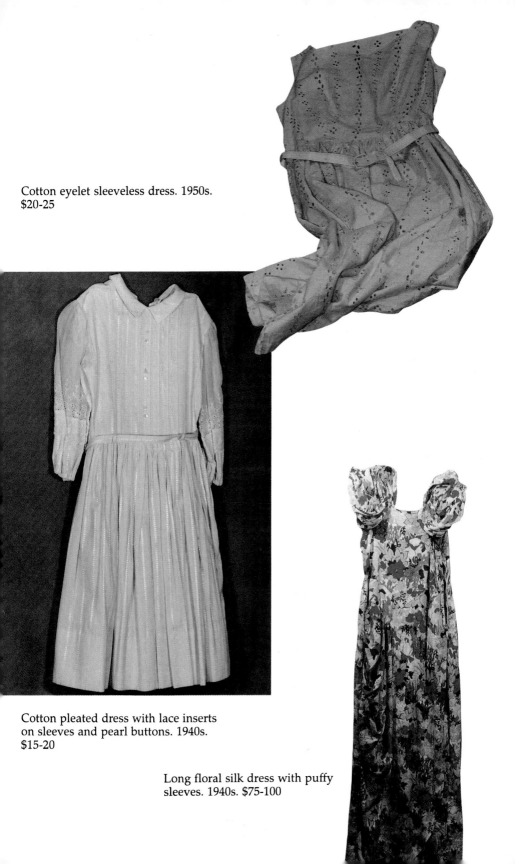

Cotton eyelet sleeveless dress. 1950s.
$20-25

Cotton pleated dress with lace inserts
on sleeves and pearl buttons. 1940s.
$15-20

Long floral silk dress with puffy
sleeves. 1940s. $75-100

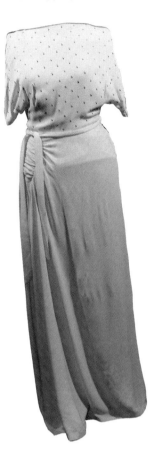

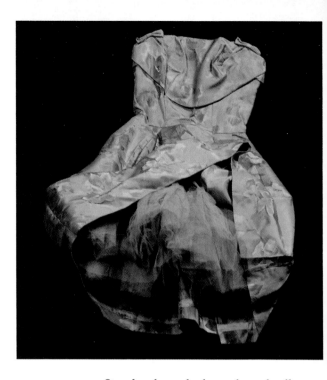

Strapless brocade dress, draped collar, with crinoline slip. 1950s. $30-40

Long evening dress with 3/4 sleeves, square neck, gathered side and rhinestone bodice. 1940s. $75-100

Crepe and nylon high waist dress trimmed in gold piping. 1950s. $30-40

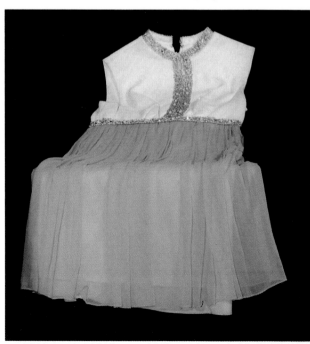

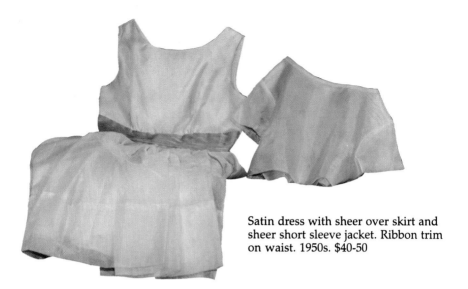

Satin dress with sheer over skirt and sheer short sleeve jacket. Ribbon trim on waist. 1950s. $40-50

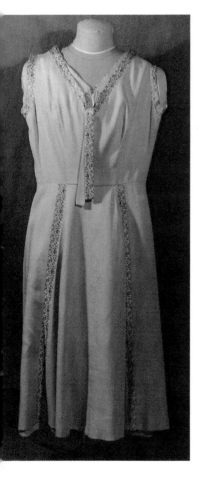

Pink linen short sleeve dress with bows on the pockets and neckline. 1940s. $30-40

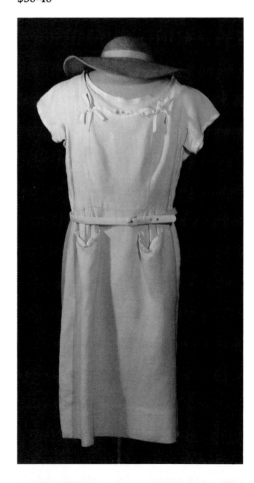

Blue linen summer dress trimmed in floral cotton. 1940s. $15-20

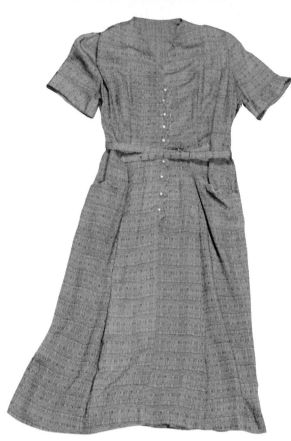

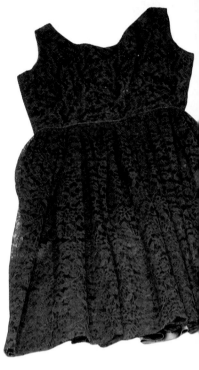

Green lace-over-silk-slip sleeveless dress. 1960s. $25-35

Nylon blend belted dress with pearlized and rhinestone buttons up the front and side pockets. 1940s. $15-20

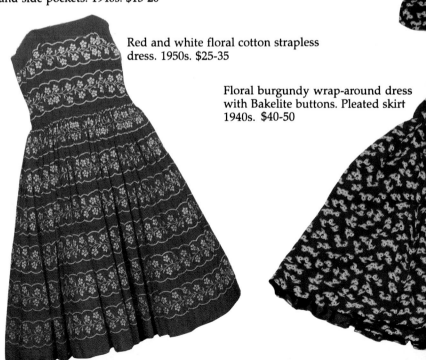

Red and white floral cotton strapless dress. 1950s. $25-35

Floral burgundy wrap-around dress with Bakelite buttons. Pleated skirt 1940s. $40-50

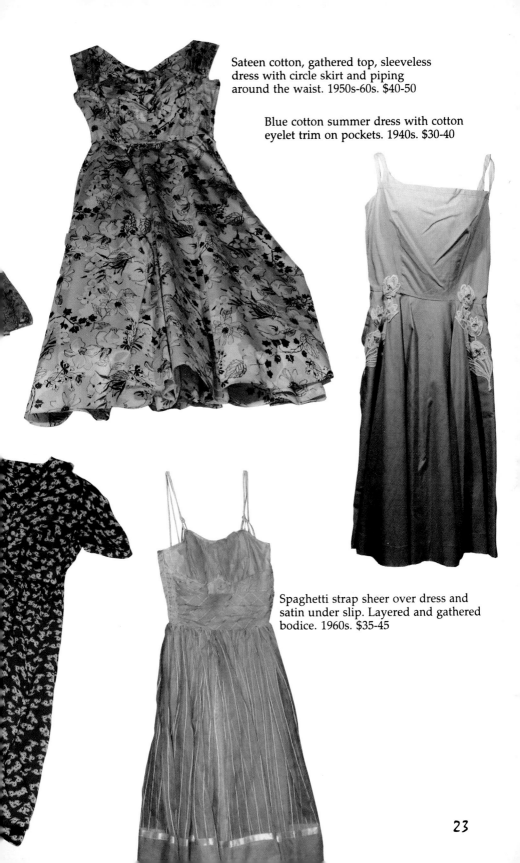

Sateen cotton, gathered top, sleeveless dress with circle skirt and piping around the waist. 1950s-60s. $40-50

Blue cotton summer dress with cotton eyelet trim on pockets. 1940s. $30-40

Spaghetti strap sheer over dress and satin under slip. Layered and gathered bodice. 1960s. $35-45

23

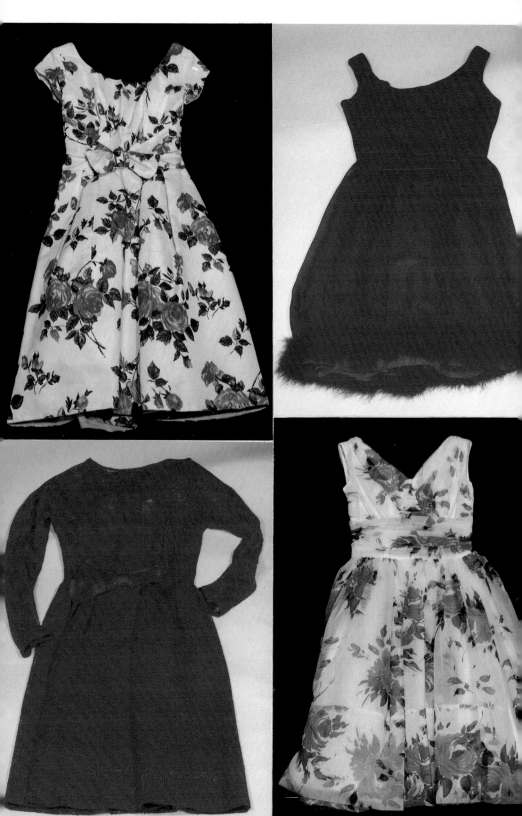

Opposite page:
Top left: Taffeta floral dress with gathered waistline and self-tie bow in front. Crinoline underslip. 1950s. $30-40

Bottom left: Satin underdress with lace overdress. 1950s. $40-50

Top right: Red sleeveless scoop neck chiffon dress with feathers decorating the bottom. 1950s-60s. $40-50

Bottom right: Sheer floral net over satin underdress. High waist. Sleeveless. 1950s. $30-40

This page:
Below: Blue satin sleeveless dress with cummerbund waist. Lace overlay and crinoline slip. 1950s. $30-40

Right: File material 3/4 sleeve print dress. Gathered waist-scoop neck. 1950s. $30-40

Bottom right: Synthetic satin-look two-piece dress. Box style double breasted jacket trimmed in pearls and rhinestones. 1950s-60s. $25-35

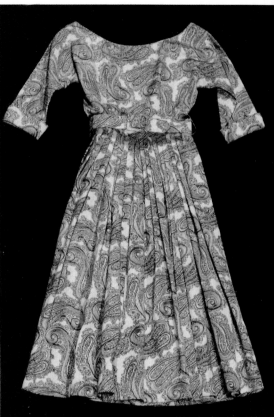

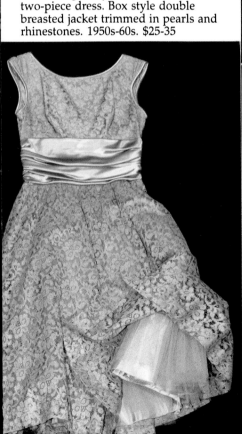

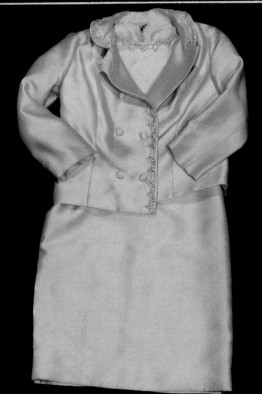

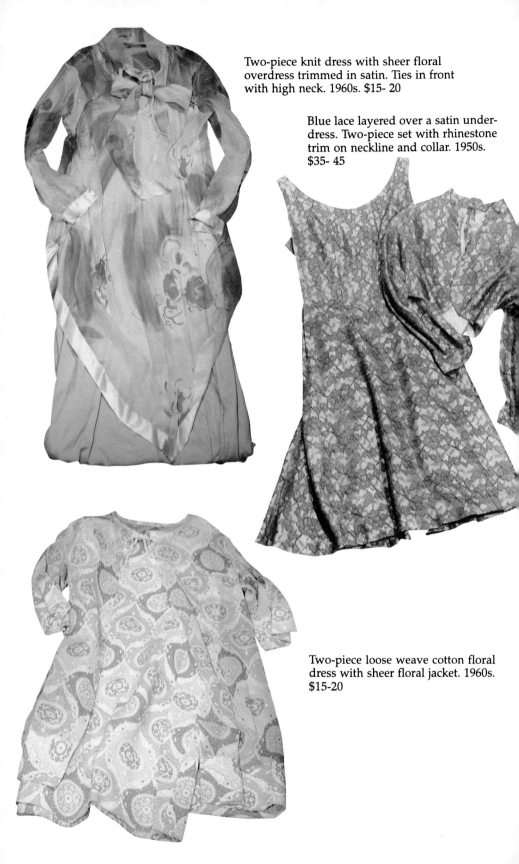

Two-piece knit dress with sheer floral overdress trimmed in satin. Ties in front with high neck. 1960s. $15- 20

Blue lace layered over a satin underdress. Two-piece set with rhinestone trim on neckline and collar. 1950s. $35- 45

Two-piece loose weave cotton floral dress with sheer floral jacket. 1960s. $15-20

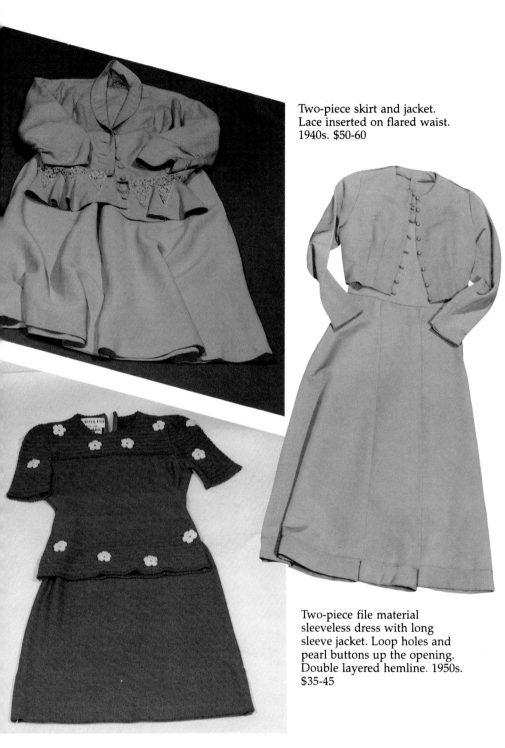

Two-piece skirt and jacket.
Lace inserted on flared waist.
1940s. $50-60

Two-piece file material
sleeveless dress with long
sleeve jacket. Loop holes and
pearl buttons up the opening.
Double layered hemline. 1950s.
$35-45

Green knit suit with crochet flower trim. 1940s.
$40-50

27

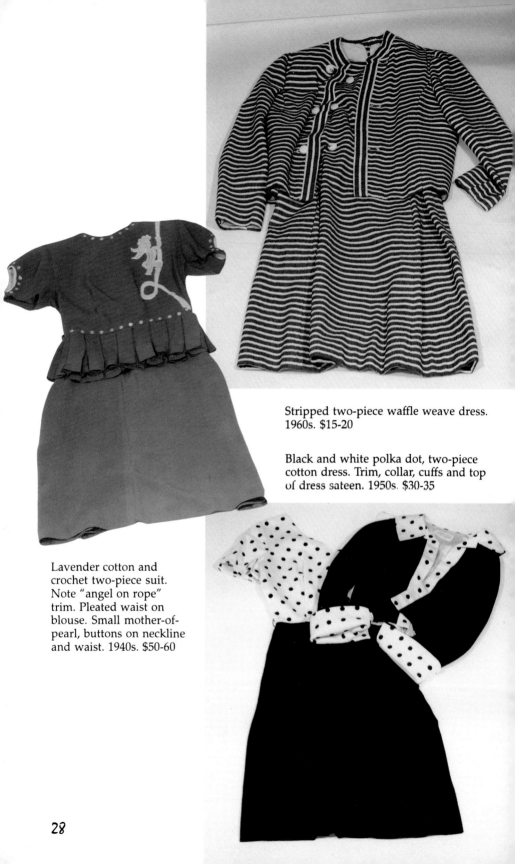

Stripped two-piece waffle weave dress. 1960s. $15-20

Black and white polka dot, two-piece cotton dress. Trim, collar, cuffs and top of dress sateen. 1950s. $30-35

Lavender cotton and crochet two-piece suit. Note "angel on rope" trim. Pleated waist on blouse. Small mother-of-pearl, buttons on neckline and waist. 1940s. $50-60

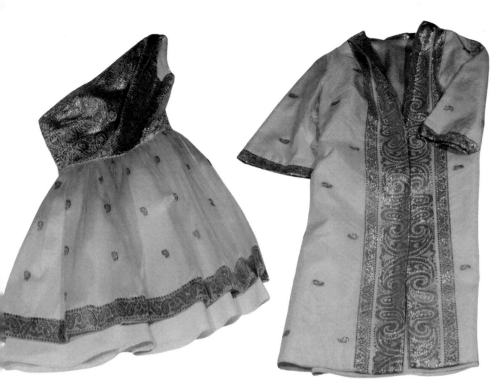

Gold Grecian dress with matching coat. 1960s. $75-100

Wide leg pant suit. Sleeveless, high waist, top trimmed in lace and a velvet ribbon. 1950s-60s. $20-30

Two-piece chiffon high waist suit. Pleated waist and pleated wide leg pants. 1950s-60s. $50-60

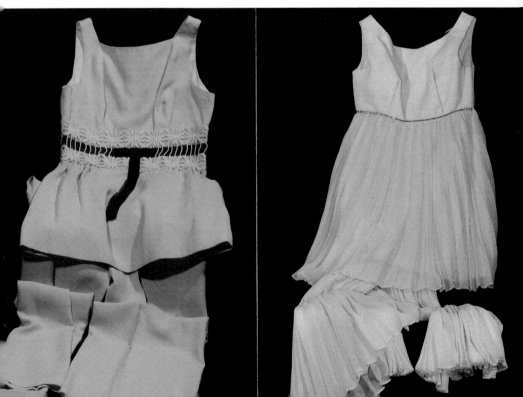

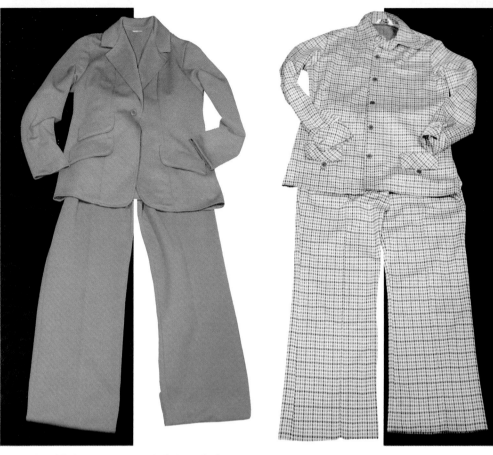

Double knit two-piece lady's wide leg
suit. 1960s- 70s. $10-15

Polyester knit two-piece lady's suit.
Wide flared legs and boxy jacket. 1960s-
70s. $10-15

Two-piece silk suit. Pleated long sleeve blouse. Small pleats in skirt front. 1960s.
$30-40

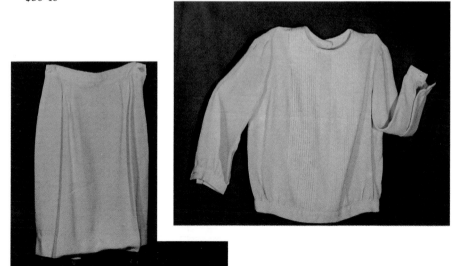

Blouses & Sweaters

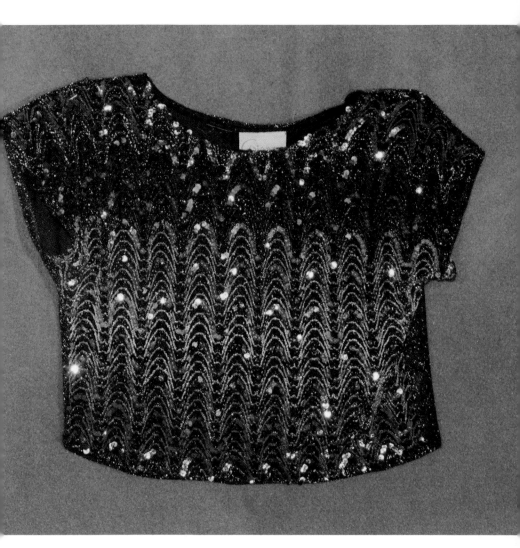

Sequined knitted cap sleeve top. 1960s. $40-50

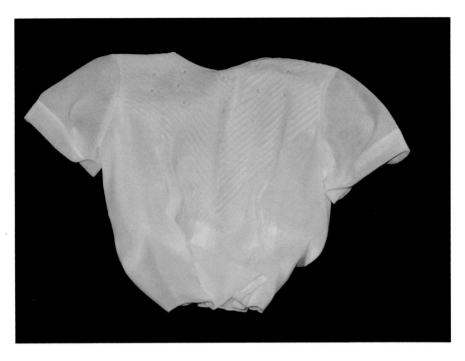

Nylon white short sleeve blouse with embroidered flowers. 1960s. $10-15

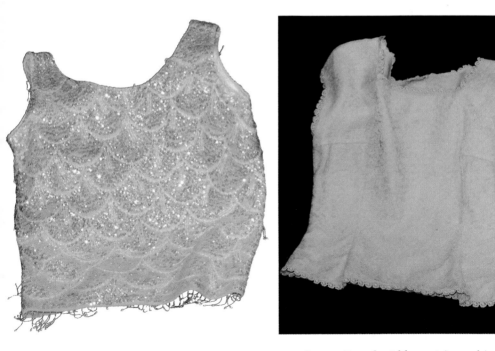

Sequined sleeveless top. 1950s. $40-50

Lace cotton short blouse trimmed in eyelet lace. 1950s. $10-15

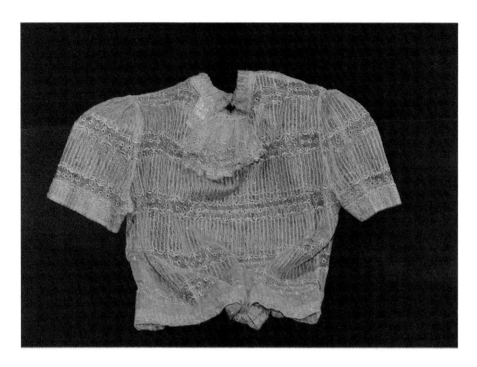

Pink, sheer lace, short sleeve blouse. 1940s. $20-30

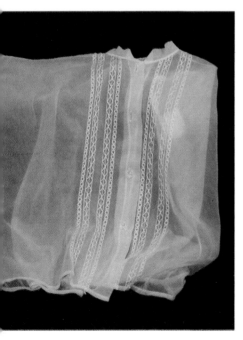

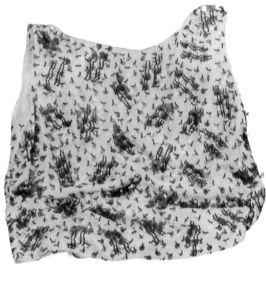

Sheer sleeveless blouse with lace trimming down the front. 1950s. $10-15

Beaded and sequined sleeveless top. 1940s. $35-40

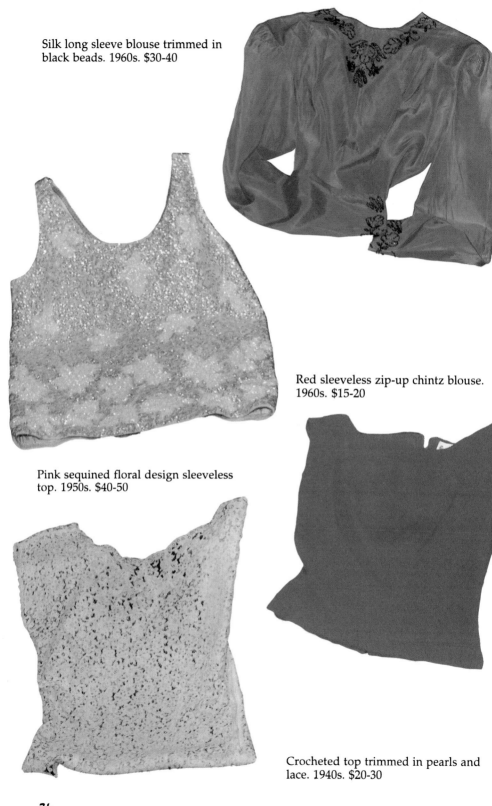

Silk long sleeve blouse trimmed in black beads. 1960s. $30-40

Red sleeveless zip-up chintz blouse. 1960s. $15-20

Pink sequined floral design sleeveless top. 1950s. $40-50

Crocheted top trimmed in pearls and lace. 1940s. $20-30

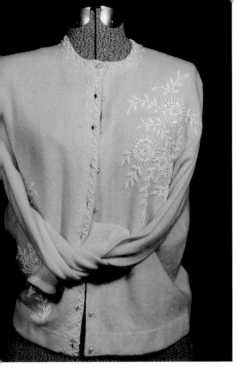

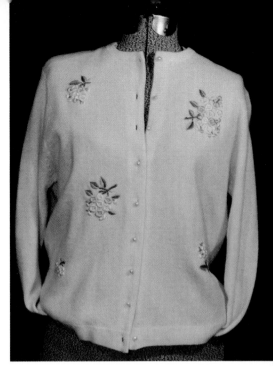

Wool sweater trimmed in beads. 1950s. $30-40

Wool sweater with appliqued flowers. 1950s. $15-20

Sequined long sleeve wool sweater with high collar. 1960s. $30-40

Gold and white beaded sweater. 1950s. $40-50

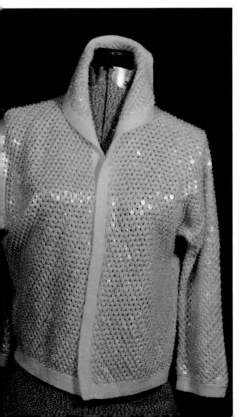

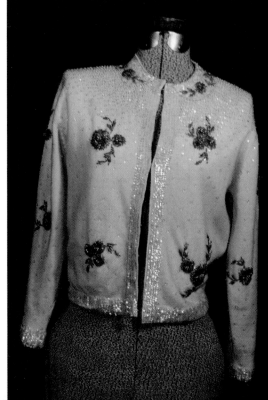

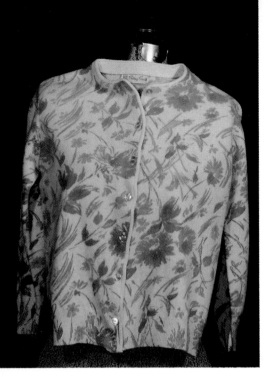

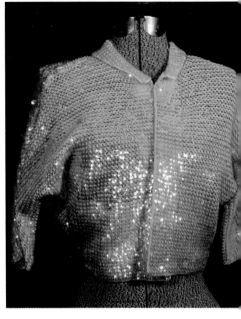

Gold flowered button-up wool sweater.1950s. $15-20

Angora and wool wild flower print sweater.1950s. $15-20

Sequined short wool sweater. 3/4 sleeves. 1960s. $30-40

Wool long sweater with wild flower print. Pull on. 1950s. $20-25

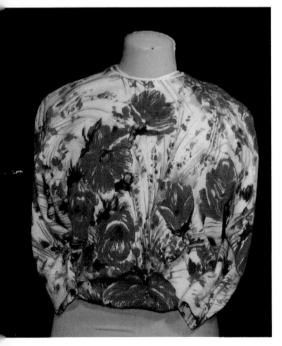

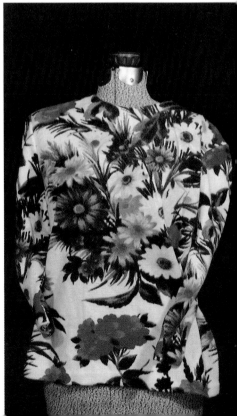

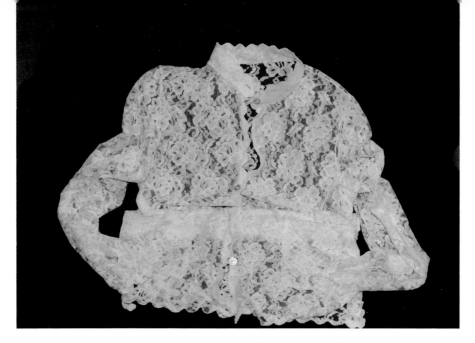

Long sleeve lace button-up blouse. 1960s. $20-30

Knitted sweater trimmed in rhinestones and pearls. 1960s. $25-30

Knitted sweater with red, white and blue cotton piping. 1960s. $15-20

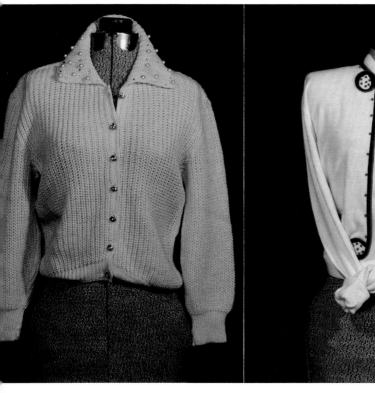

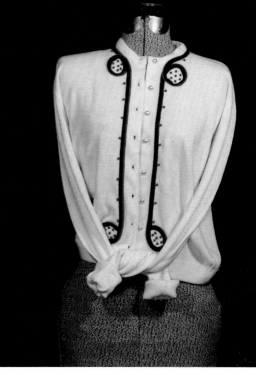

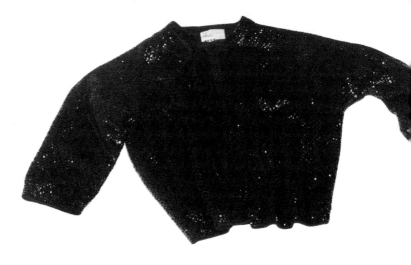

Knitted sequined jacket. 3/4 sleeves high collar. 1940s. $50-60

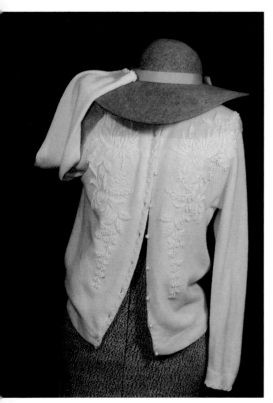

White wool beaded sweater. 1960s. $20-30

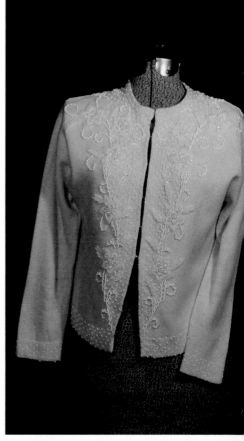

Wool beaded sweater. 1960s. $20-30

Slips & Nightwear

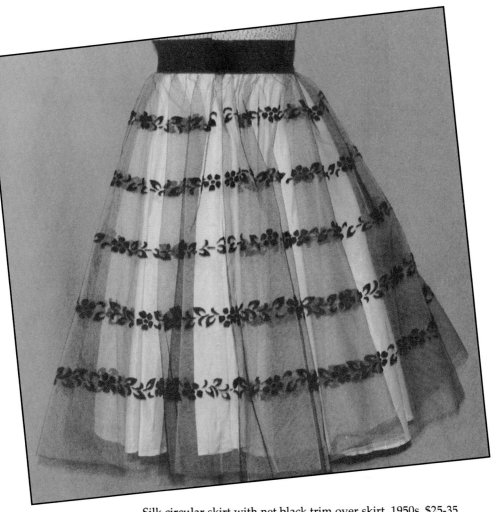

Silk circular skirt with net black trim over skirt. 1950s. $25-35

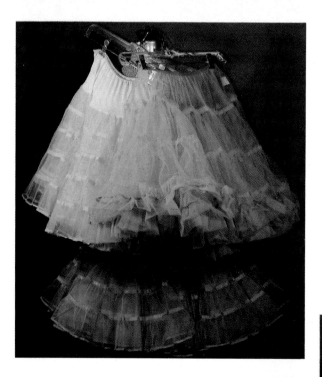

Three different colors of crinoline slips.
1950s. $20-30 each

Pink layered lace crinoline. 1950s.
$25-35

Quilted circular printed skirt. 1950s.
$20-25

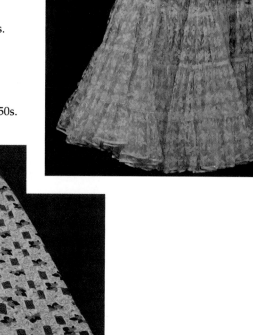

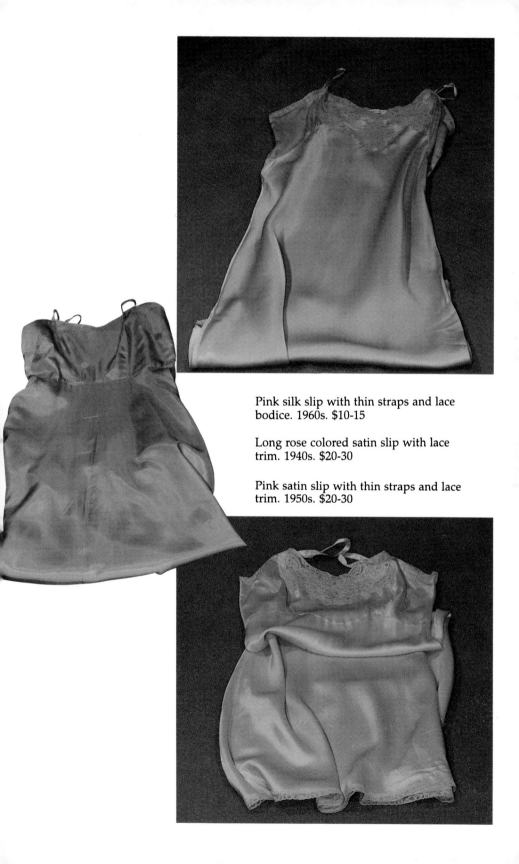

Pink silk slip with thin straps and lace bodice. 1960s. $10-15

Long rose colored satin slip with lace trim. 1940s. $20-30

Pink satin slip with thin straps and lace trim. 1950s. $20-30

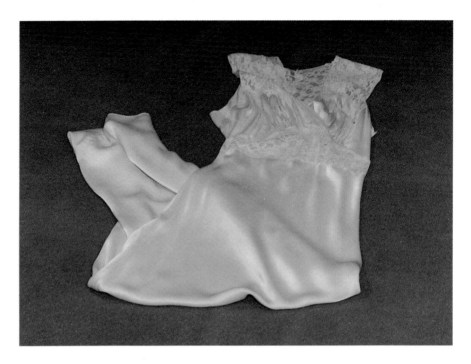

Light pink, long satin nightgown. 1960s. $25-35

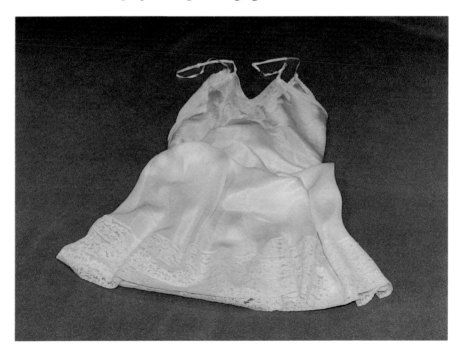

White silk slip with thin straps and layers of lace on bottom. 1960s. $20-30

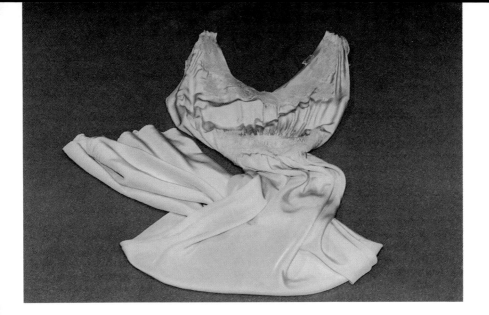

Light blue, long silk nightgown. 1950s. $20-30

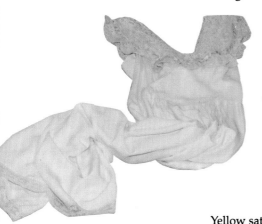

Long yellow silk nightgown with lace neckline and bottom. 1940s. $25-35

Yellow satin nightgown. Lace trim. 1940s. $25-35

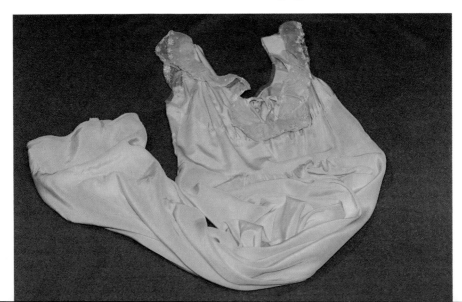

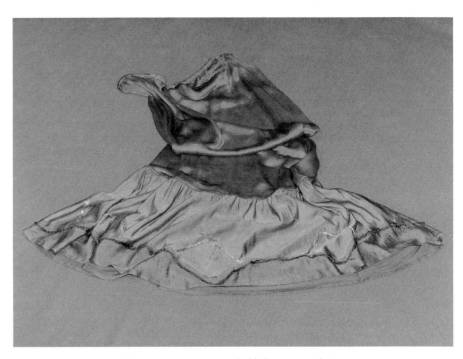

Blue and orange satin half slip. 1940s. $10-15

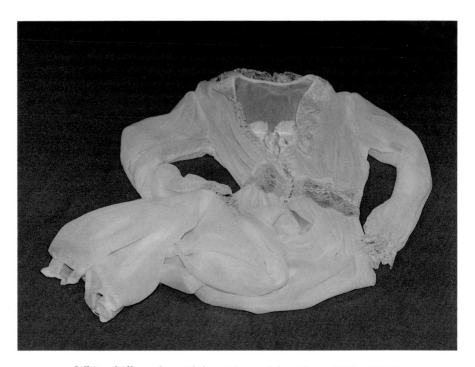

White chiffon robe with lace trim and front bow. 1950s. $30-40

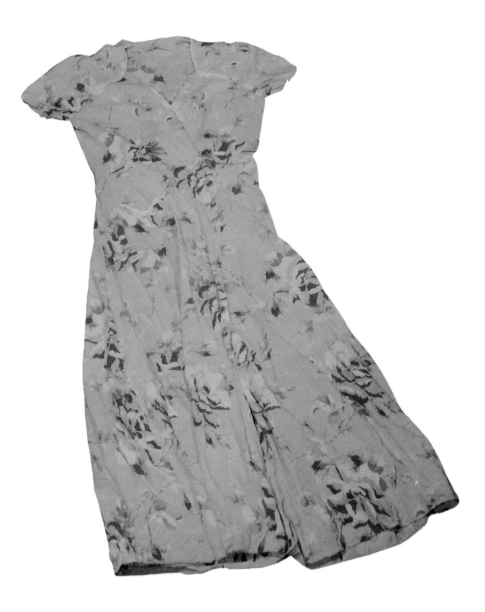

Waffle cotton floral house coat. Tie front cotton eyelet lace neckline. 1940s. $10-15

Coats

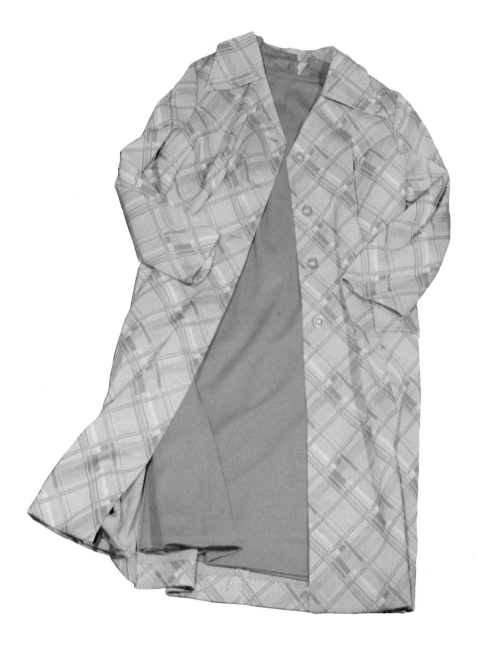

Two-piece double knit sleeveless dress and coat. Pearlized buttons on coat and zip up dress. 1950s $20-30

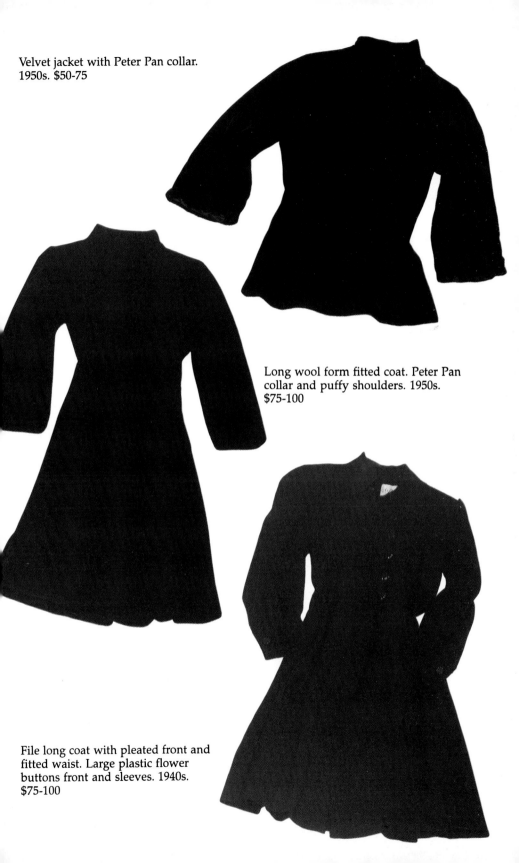

Velvet jacket with Peter Pan collar.
1950s. $50-75

Long wool form fitted coat. Peter Pan
collar and puffy shoulders. 1950s.
$75-100

File long coat with pleated front and
fitted waist. Large plastic flower
buttons front and sleeves. 1940s.
$75-100

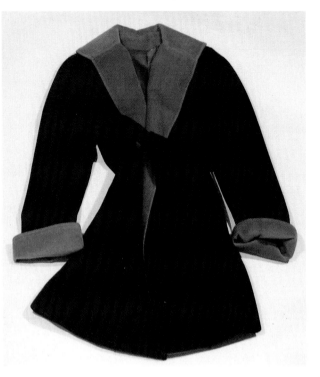

Wool black coat trimmed in brown. Ties at waist with roll up sleeves and satin lining. 1960s. $50-75

Sateen rose coat. Wide collar and large, material-covered buttons. 1950s. $30-40

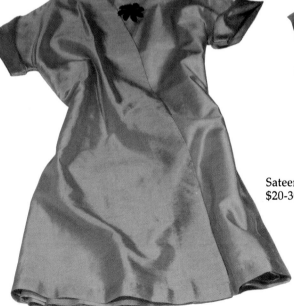

Sateen pink coat. Wide sleeves. 1950s $20-30

Plastic waffle coat with clear plastic overlay. Pleated in front. Zipper. 1950s. $30-40

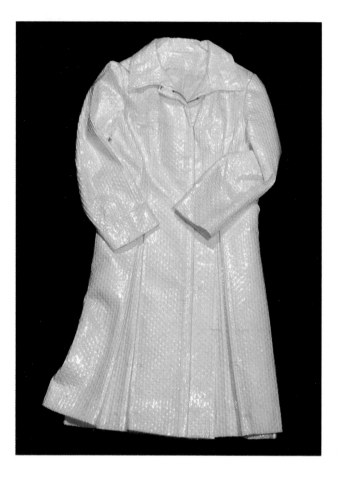

Wool brocade beaded evening jacket. Beaded front and sleeves. 1940s. $100-125

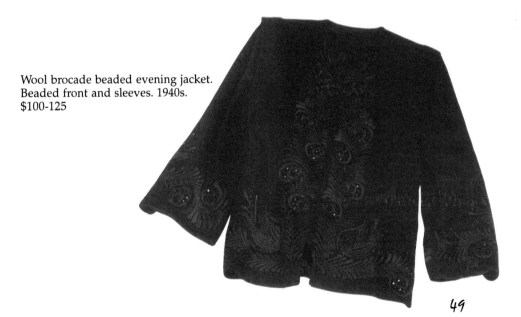

Hats

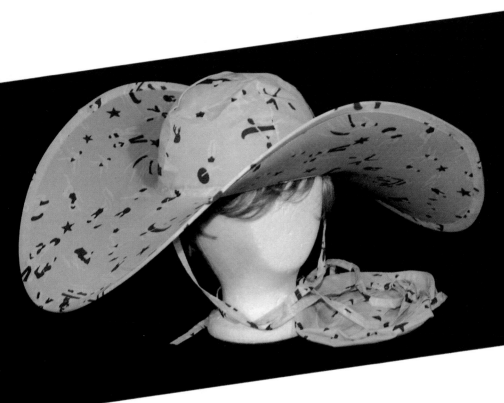

Wide brim flexible hat. Folds up and fits into a cloth bag. 1960s. $20-30

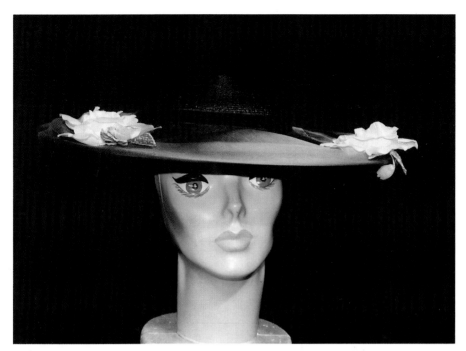

Wide brim straw hat decorated with flowers. 1940s. $25-35

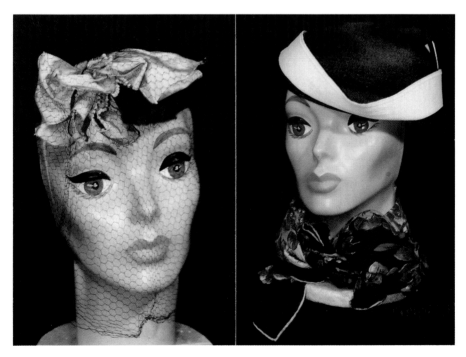

Felt netted hat with pink and blue grosgrain ribbon bows. 1940s. $20-30

Navy straw hat with white brim. 1940s. $12-15

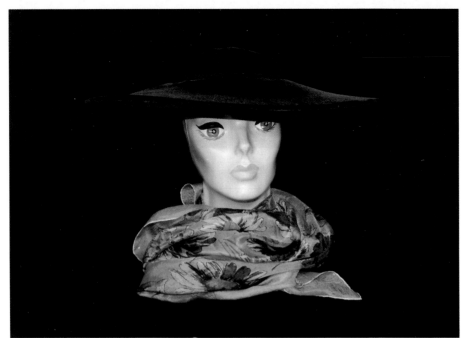

Navy wide brim straw hat. 1940s. $25-35

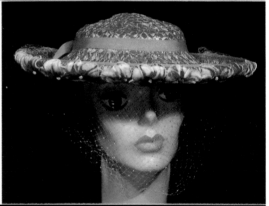

Wide brim straw hat with netting. 1960s. $20-25

Black straw rounded hat decorated with daisies. 1940s. $30-40

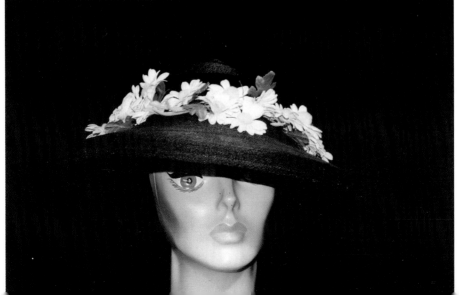

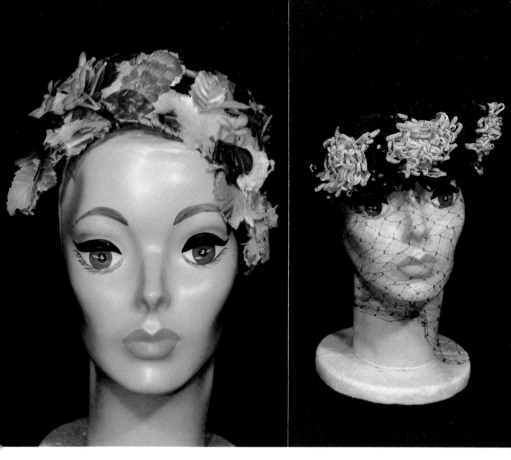

Floral and leaf hat. 1960s. $8-12

Black felt hat with flowers and netting. 1940s. $30-40

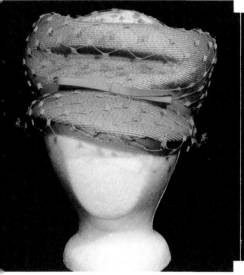

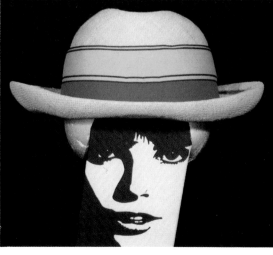

Straw hat with bow in front and netting. 1950s. $15-20

Sacks Fifth Avenue straw hat trimmed in colorful grosgrain ribbon. 1950s. $20-25

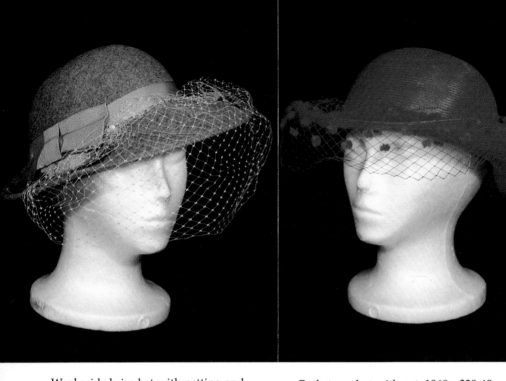

Wool wide brim hat with netting and grosgrain ribbon trim. 1950s. $35-45

Red straw hat with net. 1960s. $30-40

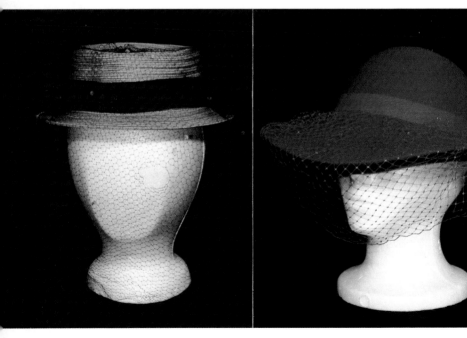

Straw hat with ribbon trim and netting. 1950s. $15- 20

Wool wide brim hat with netting. 1950s. $30-40

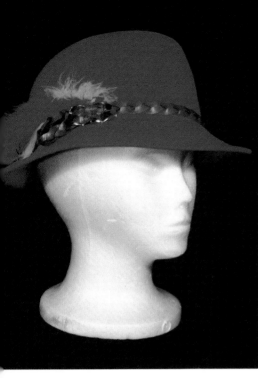

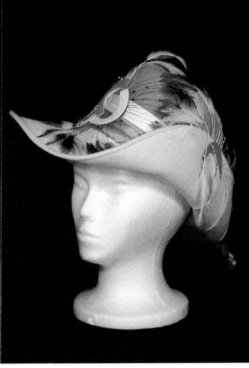

Red wool hat with leather trim and feather. 1960s. $30-40

Curved wool hat with pheasant feathers and ribbon trim. 1960s. $35-45

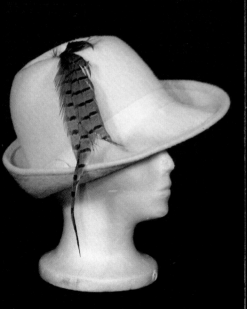

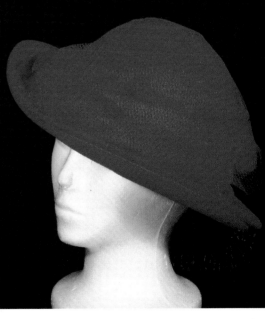

Wool hat with feather and ribbon trim. 1950s. $30- 40

Wool curved brim hat with net. 1950s. $35-45

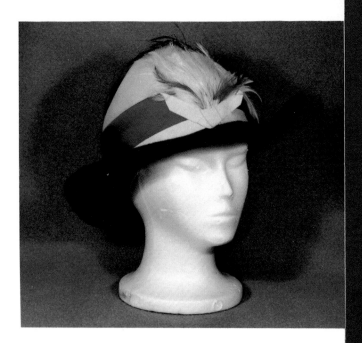

Black wool hat with feather decoration
in front. 1960s. $30-40

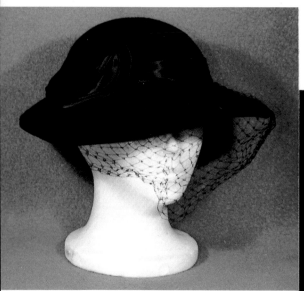

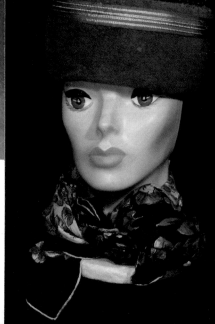

Black doe skin hat with silk flower and
netting. 1940s. $30-40

Felt pill box hat with ribbon trim and
netting. 1950s. $10-15

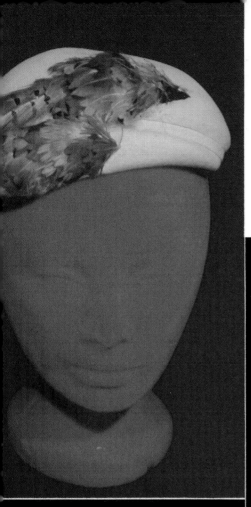

Wool hat decorated with a pheasant feather. 1940s. $15-20

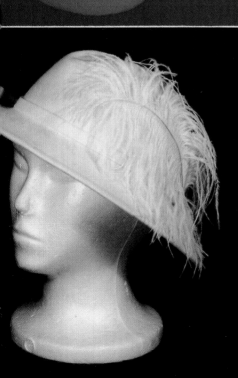

Wool hat decorated with feather. 1950s. $30-40

Wool curved brim hat decorated with feathers. 1950s. $30-40

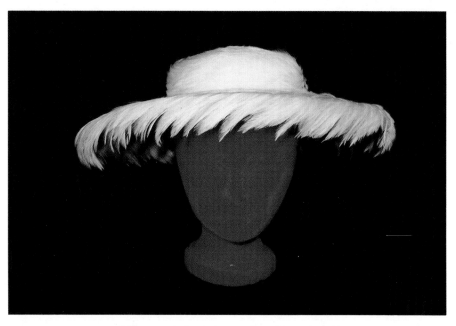

White wide brim feather hat. 1950s. $40-50

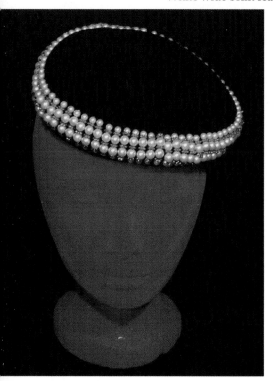

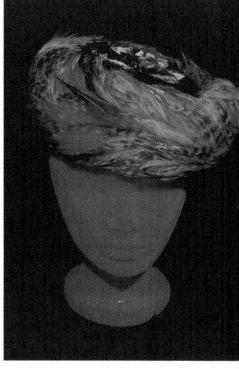

Velvet hat decorated with beads. 1940s. $15-20

Pheasant feather hat. 1940s. $25-30

58

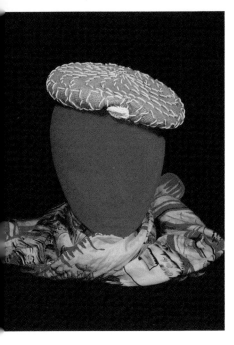

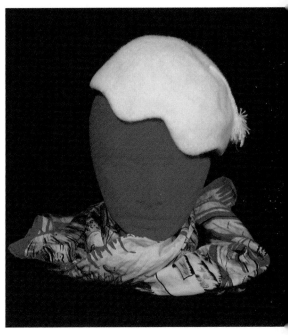

Beaded felt cap. 1940s. $10-15

White wool hat with feather decoration.
1940s. $10- 15

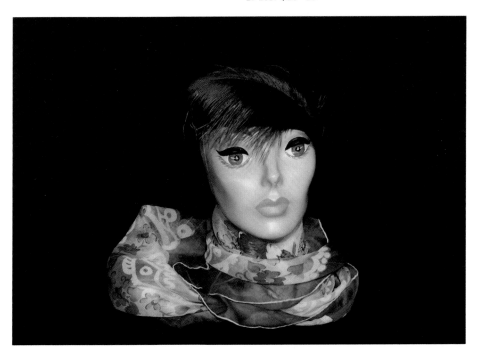

Brown felt and feather hat. 1940s. $20-25

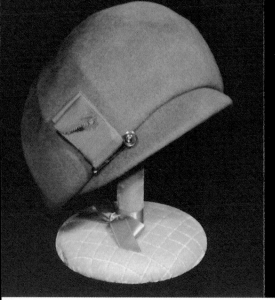

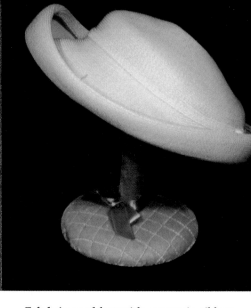

Wool cap trimmed with ribbon and a hat clip. 1940s. $15-20

Felt brimmed hat with grosgrain ribbon trim. 1940s. $20-25

Satin hat with netting. 1950s. $8-12

Leopard look cap. 1950s. $10-15

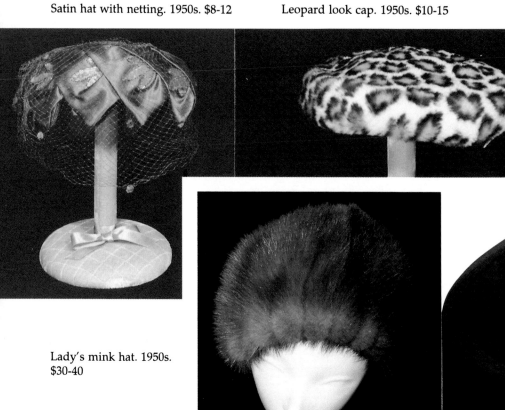

Lady's mink hat. 1950s.
$30-40

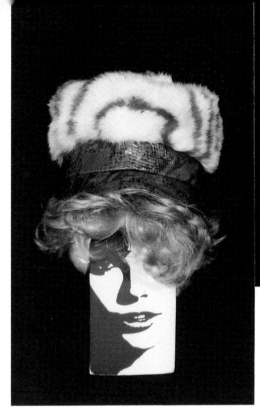

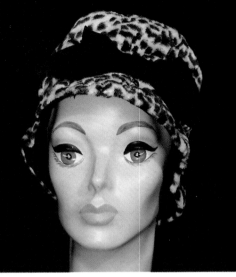

Imitation leopard pill box hat with velvet bow. 1950s. $10-15

Groovy fur and leather cap. 1960s. $20-25

Wide brim hat decorated with ribbon and flower. 1940s. $30-40

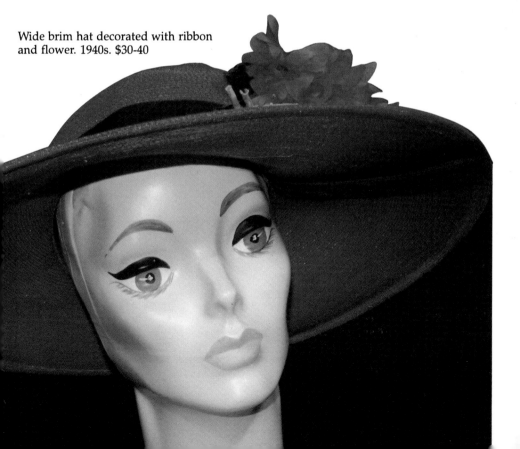

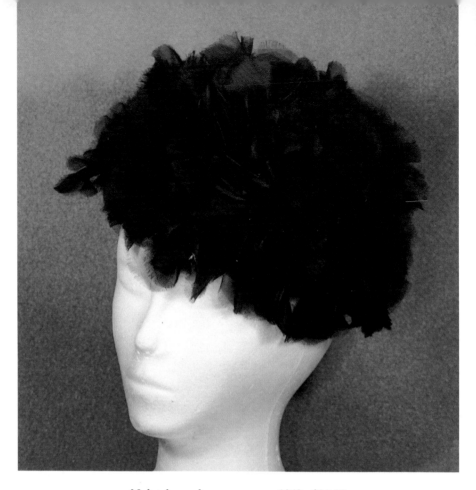

Nylon bowed cover-up cap. 1960s. $20-30

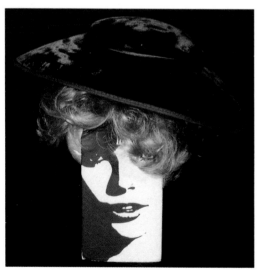

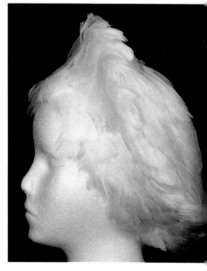

Brown velvet netted hat. 1940s. $15-20   White feather stretch tam. 1940s. $40-50

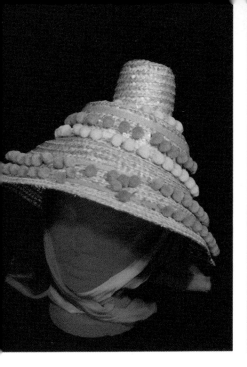

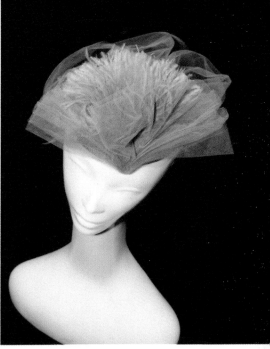

Chenille tasseled straw summer hat. 1960s. $5-8

Lady's felt hat decorated in feathers and net. 1940s. $10-15

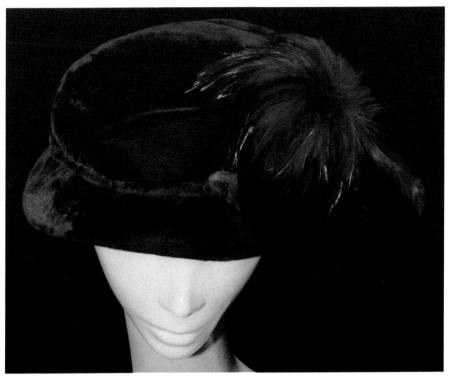

Lady's velvet hat with brim and feather trim. 1940s. $10-15

Shoes

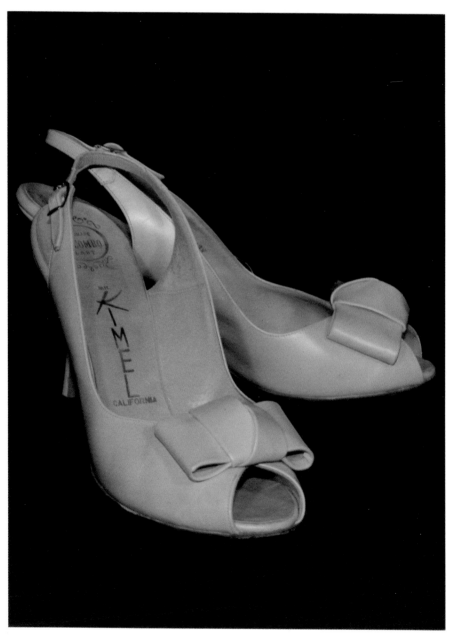

Cream back strap toeless high heel shoes with bow trim. 1950s. $20-30

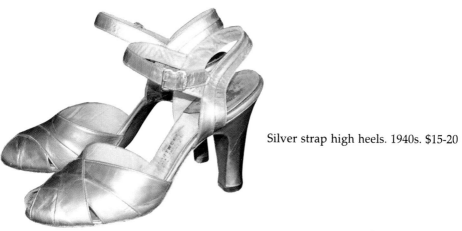

Silver strap high heels. 1940s. $15-20

Silver strap wide heel shoes. 1940s. $10-15

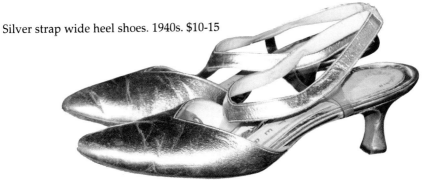

Silver front strap low heels with beige leather trim. 1940s. $10-15

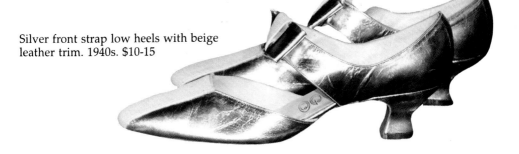

Low heel back strap shoes. 1940s. $15-20

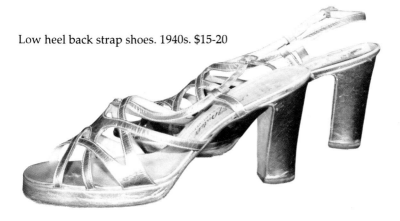

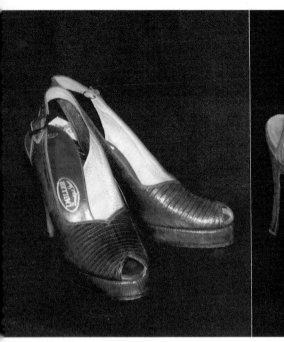
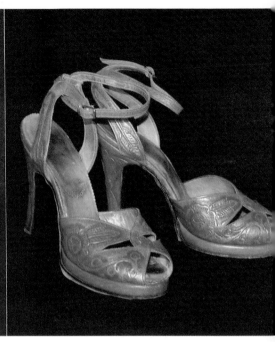

Brown lizard, open-toed platform
shoes. 1940s. $50-60

Hand-tooled ankle strap platform
shoes. 1940s. $50-60

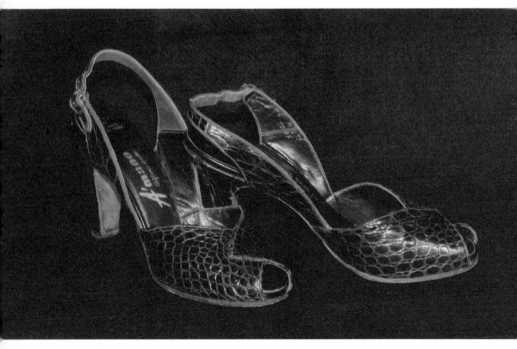

Alligator slingback, open-toe shoes. 1950s. $40-50

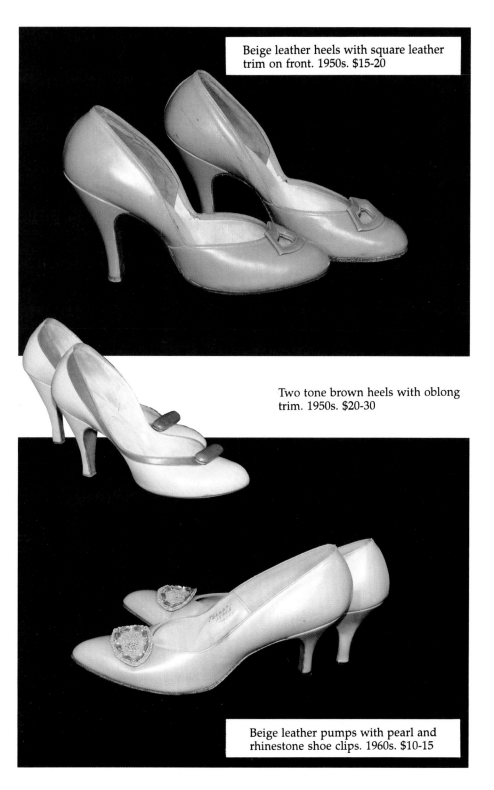

Beige leather heels with square leather trim on front. 1950s. $15-20

Two tone brown heels with oblong trim. 1950s. $20-30

Beige leather pumps with pearl and rhinestone shoe clips. 1960s. $10-15

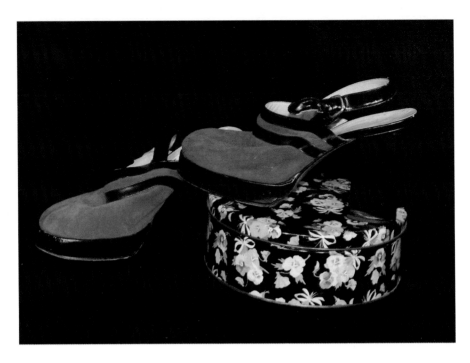

Red suede shoes with black leather heels and trim. 1960s. $20-30

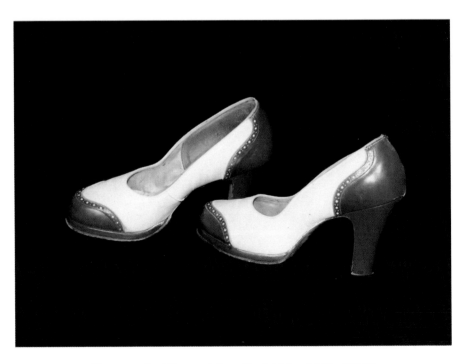

Brown and white spectators. Eyelet trim. 1940s. $20-30

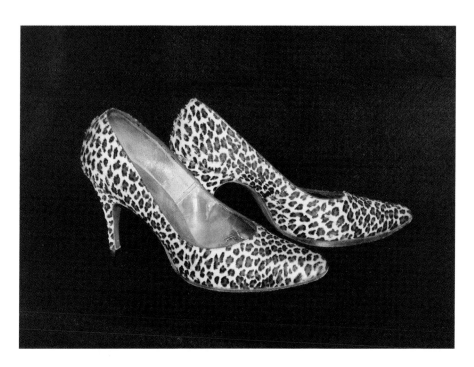

Leopard high heels. 1950s. $40-50

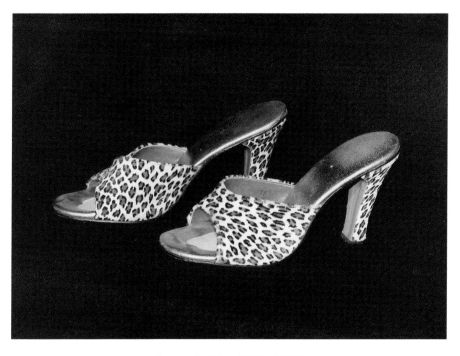

Leopard slides. 1950s. $45-55

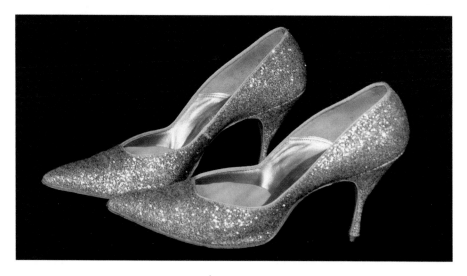

Gold glitter spike heels. 1950s. $45-55

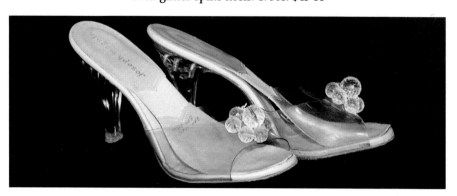

Lucite slides with lucite beads trimming the toes. 1950s. $20-30

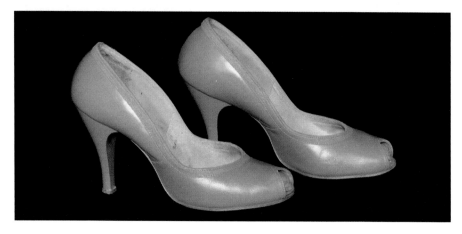

Pink open-toed high heels. 1940s. $30-40

Purses

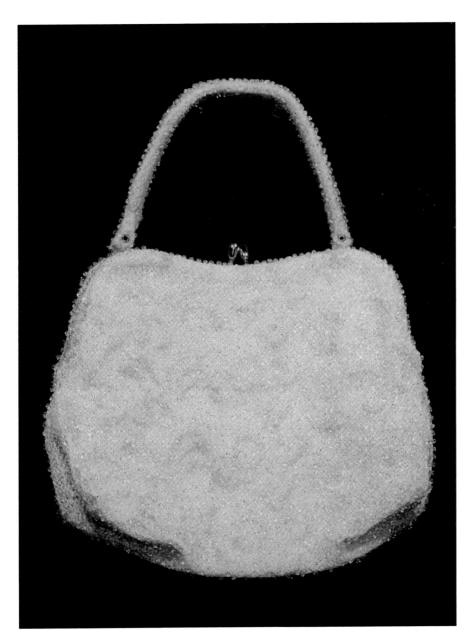

Embroidered purse with plastic beads and matching handle. Gold-tone clasp. 1940s.
$40-50

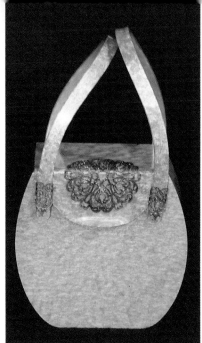

Lucite purse with gold-tone lace
decorations. 1940s. $50-65

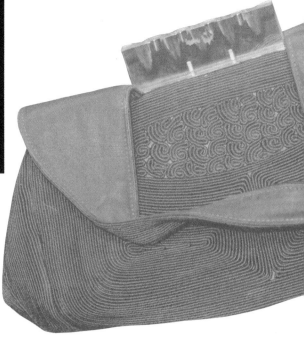

Cotton cord handbag with plastic closure. 1940s. $40-50

Cloth purse with plastic handle. 1940s. $35-45

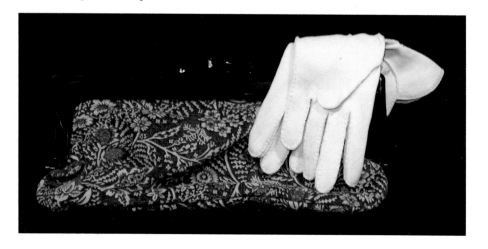

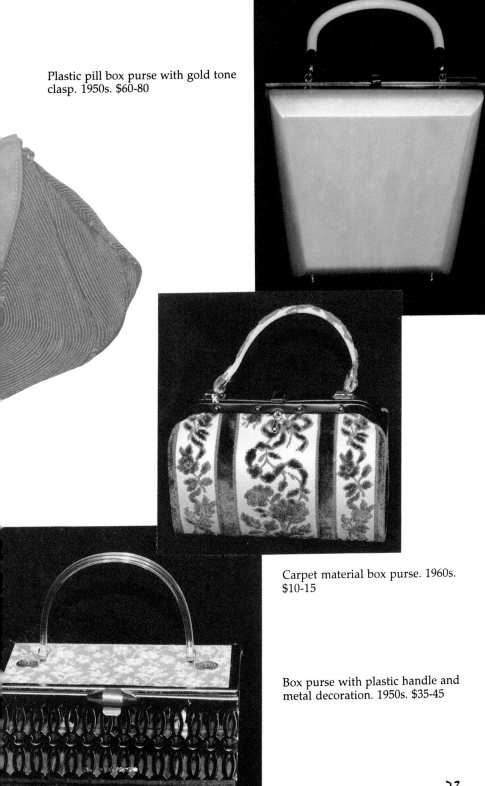

Plastic pill box purse with gold tone clasp. 1950s. $60-80

Carpet material box purse. 1960s. $10-15

Box purse with plastic handle and metal decoration. 1950s. $35-45

73

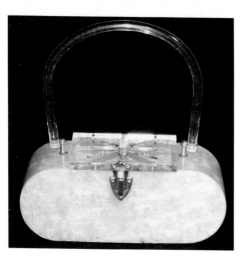

Lucite pill box purse. 1940s. $60-75

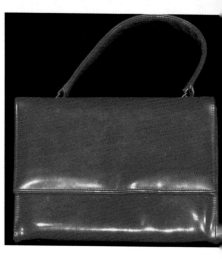

Patent leather purse. 1960s. $10-15

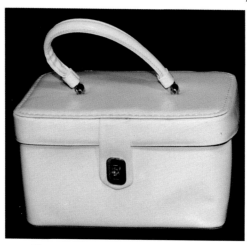

Plastic box style purse. 1950s. $15-20

Lucite purse. 1940s. $70-90

Confetti plastic pill box purse. Gold-tone hinge. 1940s. $60-75

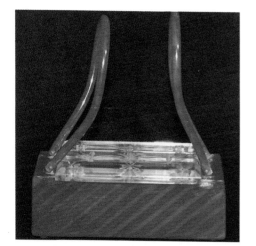

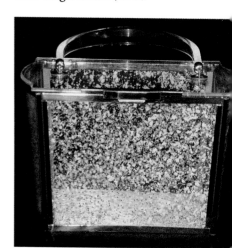

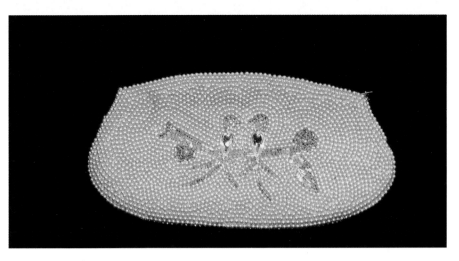

Clutch with cream colored plastic beads and rhinestones. 1940s. $30-40

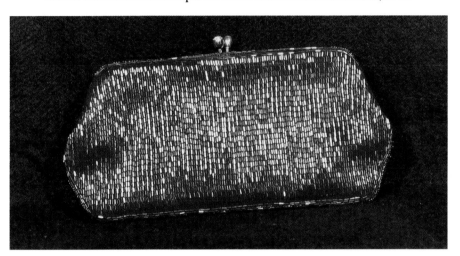

Cobalt blue glass beads cover this clutch bag. 1940s. $40- 50

Plastic beaded clutch bag. "Davis Import." 1940s. $35-45

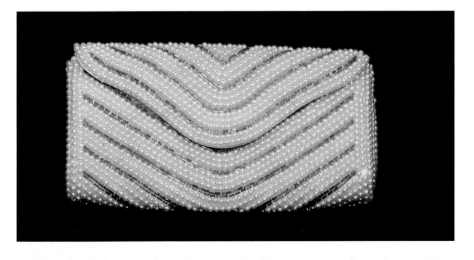

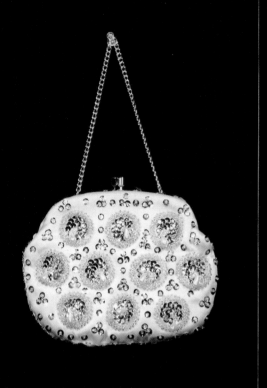

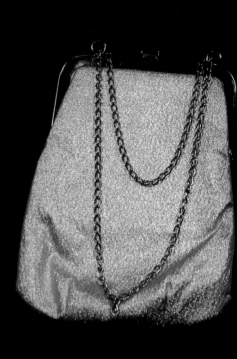

Gold vinyl purse with chain handle and plastic frame. 1950s. $15-20

Silk purse with sequins, pearls, and a chain handle. Hong Kong/China. 1950s. $20-30

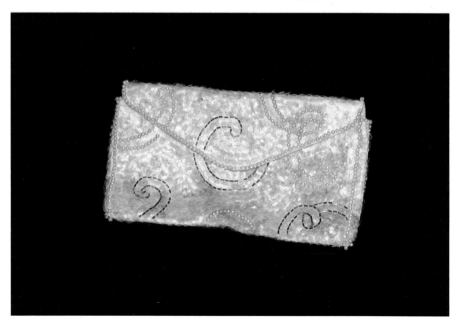

Sequined clutch bag. 1960s. $8-12

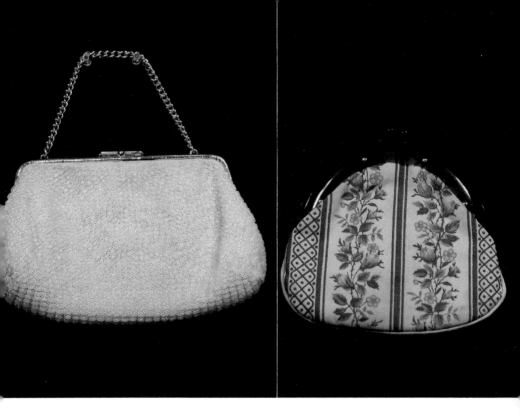

Purse with aqua plastic beads and gold-tone clasp. Reversible to pink. 1950s. $35-45

Cotton clutch bag with tortoise shell handle. 1950s. $25-30

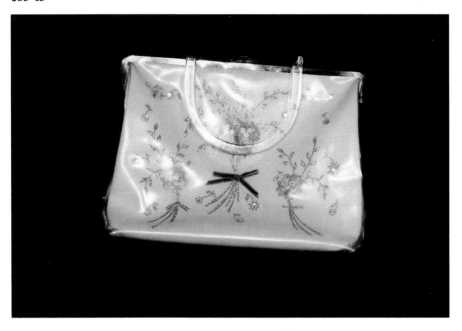

Clear plastic over floral cotton purse with plastic handle. 1960s. $10-15

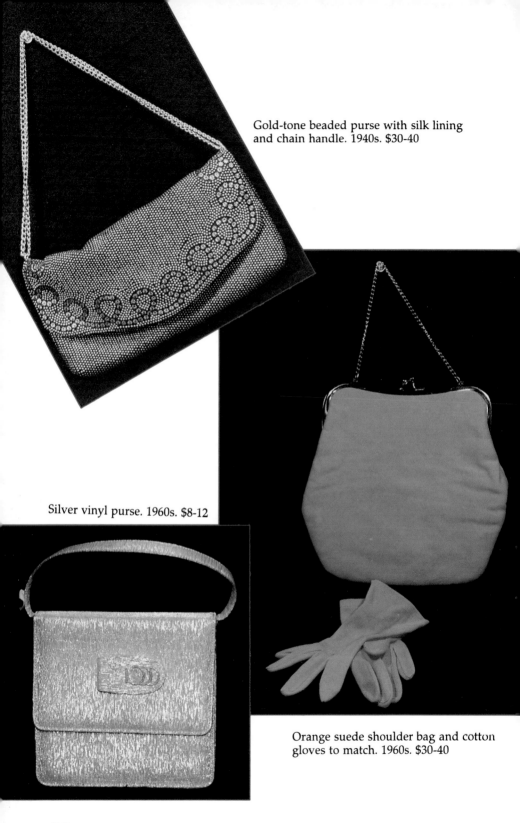

Gold-tone beaded purse with silk lining and chain handle. 1940s. $30-40

Silver vinyl purse. 1960s. $8-12

Orange suede shoulder bag and cotton gloves to match. 1960s. $30-40

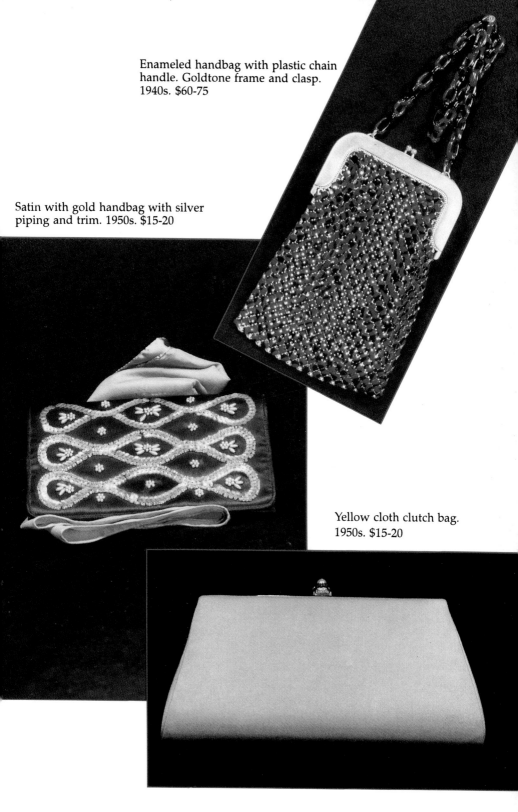

Enameled handbag with plastic chain handle. Goldtone frame and clasp. 1940s. $60-75

Satin with gold handbag with silver piping and trim. 1950s. $15-20

Yellow cloth clutch bag. 1950s. $15-20

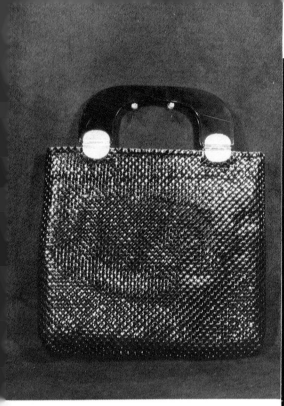

Black enamel handbag with tortoise
shell handle. "La Regale." 1940s. $30-40

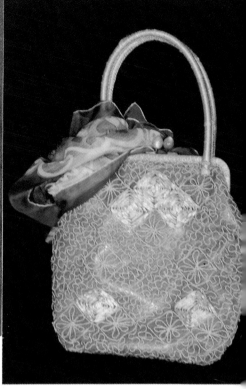

Straw purse with plastic under lining.
1950s. $10-15

Suede and leather hand- tooled purse.
1950s. $20-30

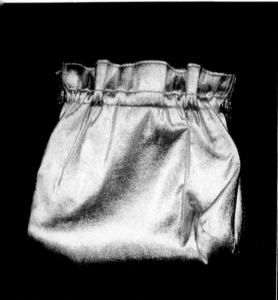

Gold lame pull string purse. 1950s.
$15-20

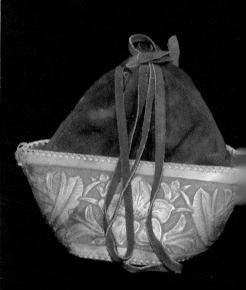

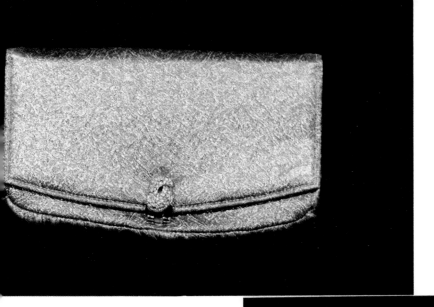

Gold brocade clutch bag. 1950s. $20-30

Silk purse with sequins, drop beads, and chain handle. 1960s. $15-20

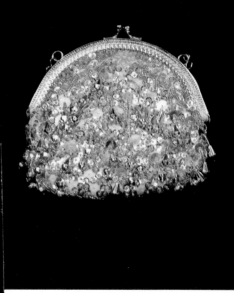

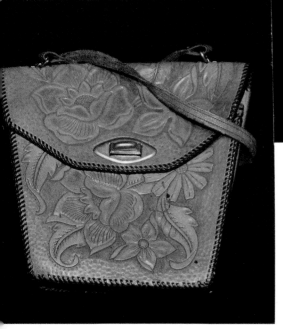

Hand tooled leather purse. 1950s. $25-30

81

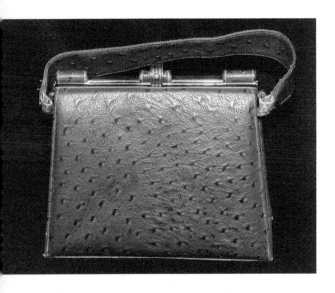

Three-way handbag. Extra strap for clutch bag and longer strap for shoulder bag. 1960s. $15-20

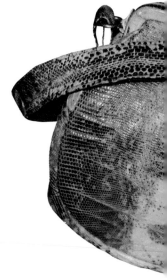

Snake skin purse. 1960s. $20-25

Alligator purse. 1960s. $25-35

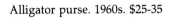

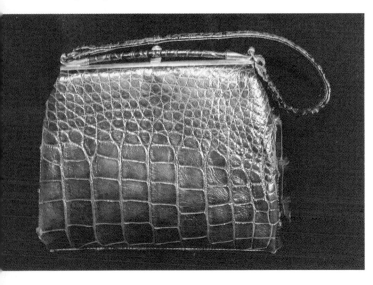

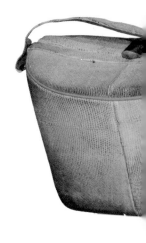

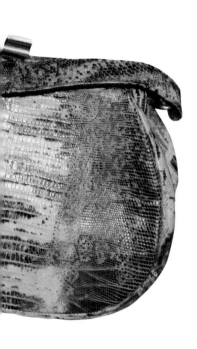

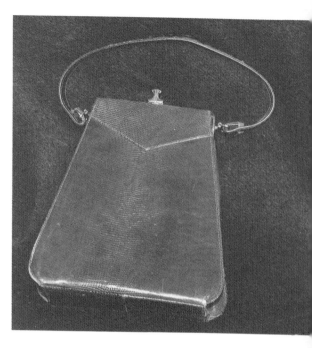

Tall lizard handbag. 1960s. $30-40

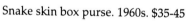

Snake skin box purse. 1960s. $35-45

Alligator clutch bag. 1960s. $20-30

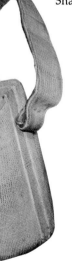

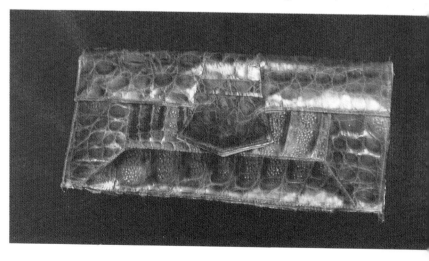

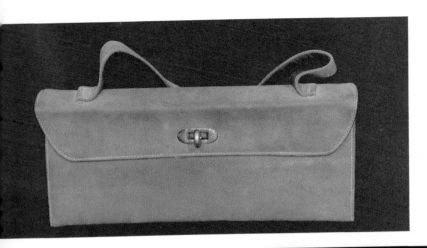

Brown suede purse. 1960s. $15-20

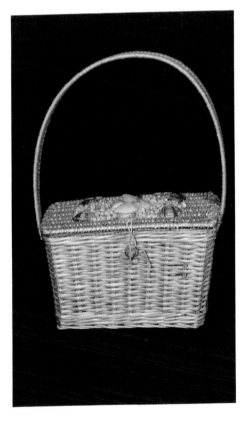

Black leather handbag with plastic handle. 1950s. $30-40

Wicker basket purse. 1960s. $8-12

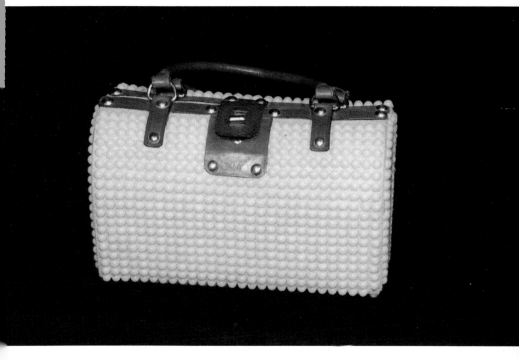

Plastic bead-look purse with leather handle. 1950s. $20-25

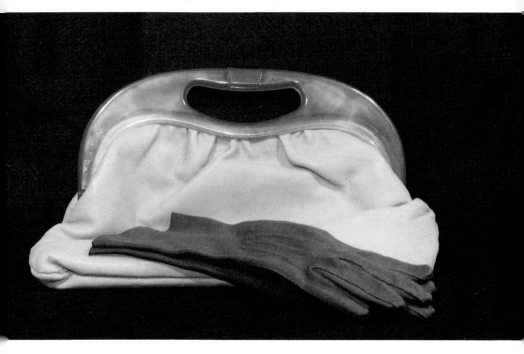

Kid skin clutch bag with tortoise shell handle. 1940s. $40-50

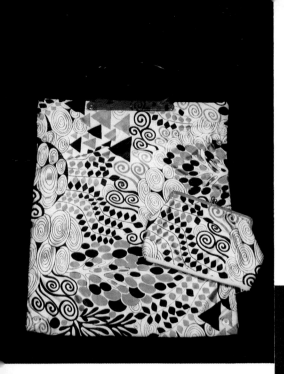

Satin lined bag with plastic handle, silk material, and a small matching change purse. 1960s. $10-15

Plastic black and white checkered cosmetic case. 1950s. $10-15

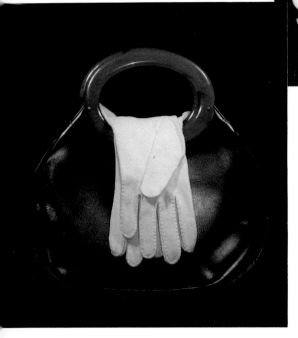

Black leather purse with tortoise shell handle. 1950s. $35-45

Scarves

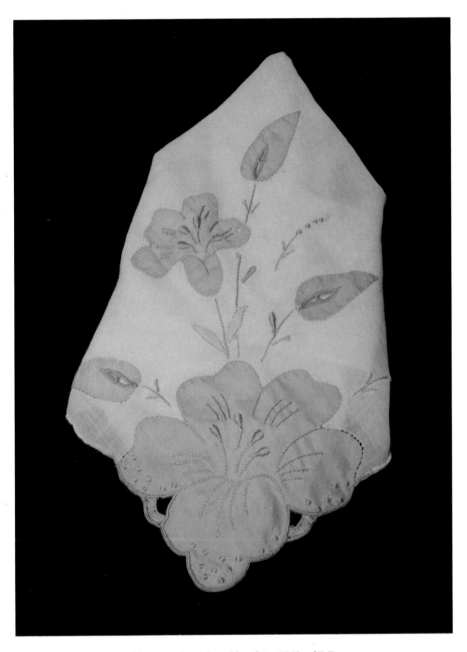

Linen embroidered hankie. 1960s. $5-7

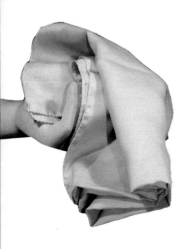

Light aqua silk scarf from Italy. 1950s. $10-15

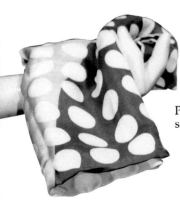

Polka dot brown and aqua silk scarf signed "Echo." 1960s. $15-20

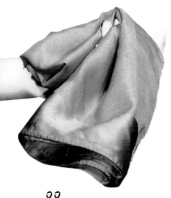

Silk neck scarf. 1950s. $8-12

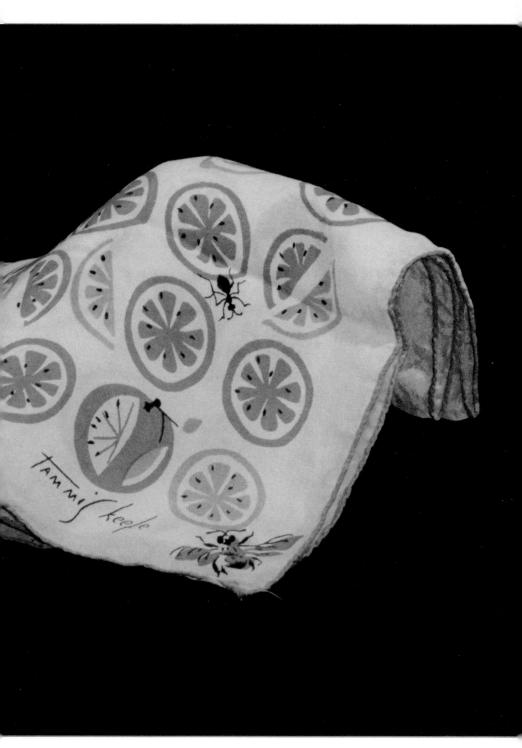

Silk scarf signed "Tammi Skeef." 1950s. $15-20

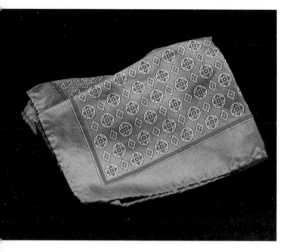

Man's ascot silk scarf. 1950s. $8-12

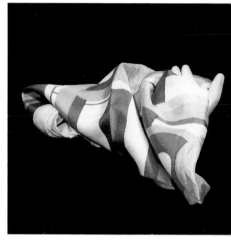

Water repellent silk scarf. 1960s. $10-15

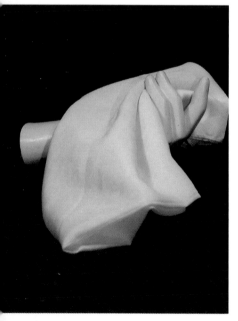

Pink polyester scarf from Italy. 1960s. $10-15

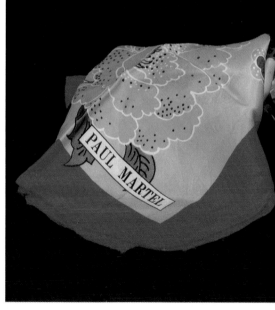

Multi-colored designer silk scarf, signed "Paul Martel." 1960s. $15-20

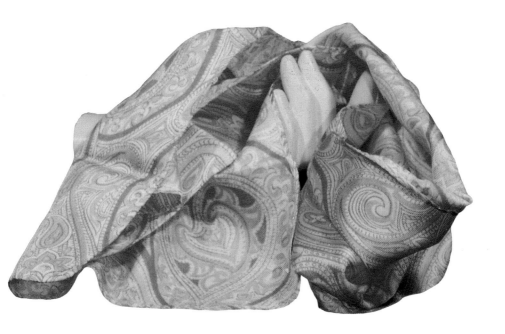

Orange paisley silk scarf. 1960s. $15-20

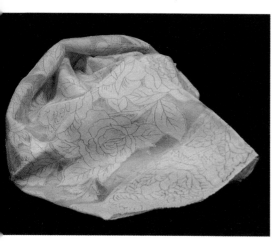

Sheer silk with floral pattern. 1960s. $15-20

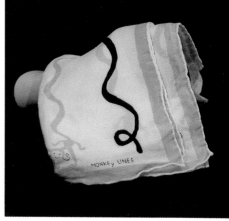

Hand-made designer silk scarf, signed "Monkey Lines." 1950s. $20-25

Gloves

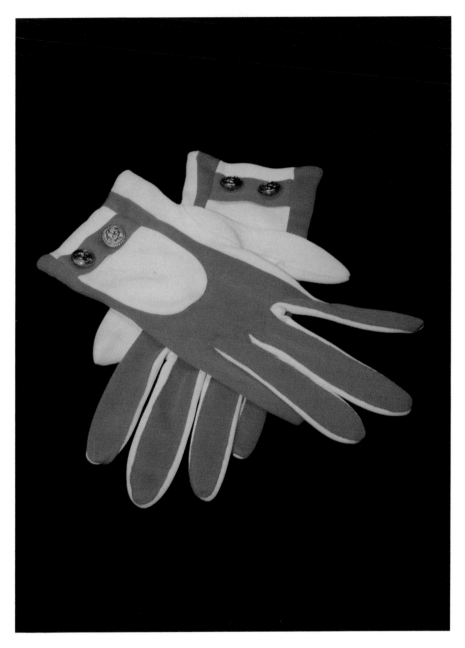

Lady's cotton gloves with metal button trim. 1960s. $10-15

Red leather lady's gloves. 1950s. $15-20

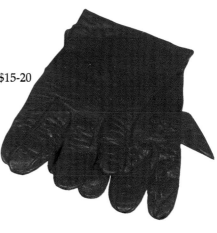

Pink double woven "Fownes" gloves decorated with pearl buttons. 1950s. $10-15

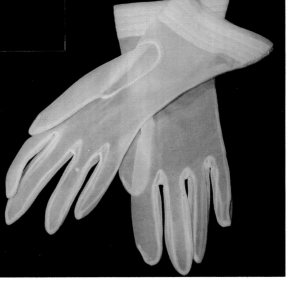

Lady's sheer gloves. Wrist has widened double fold trim. 1950s. $10-15

Cotton gloves by K. Sekl. 1950s. $15-20

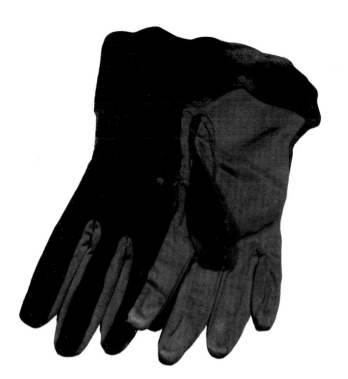

Black lady's velvet and silk gloves.
U.S.A. 1950s. $10-15

Brown English cotton, double woven
gloves. 1950s. $8-12

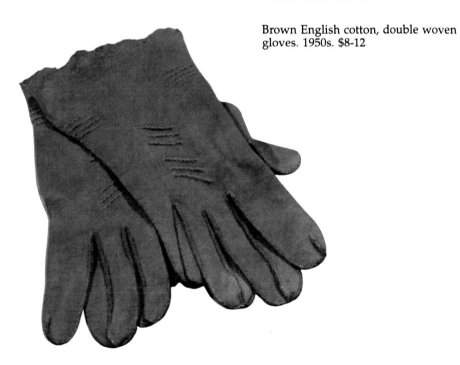

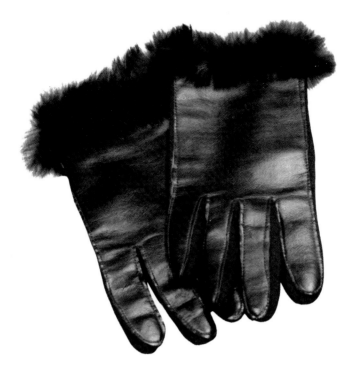

Black leather and fur gloves. 1940s.
$15-20

Brown cotton suede gloves from Italy.
1960s. $15- 20

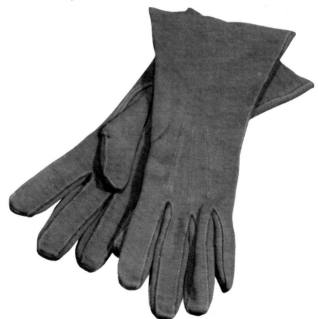

Sunglasses

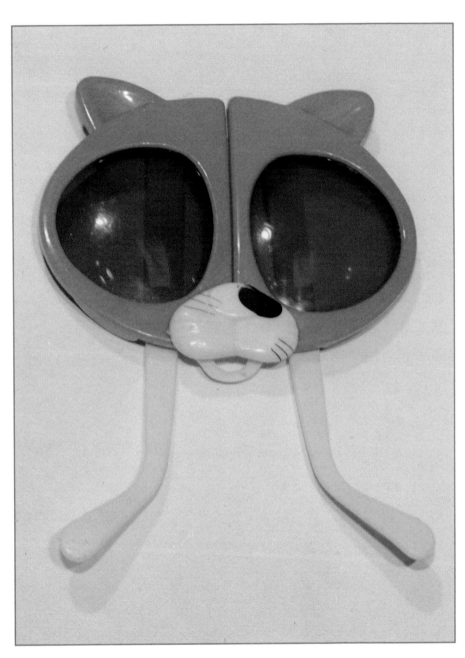

Plastic cat sunglasses. Folded. Opens up for regular glasses. 1960s. $10-15

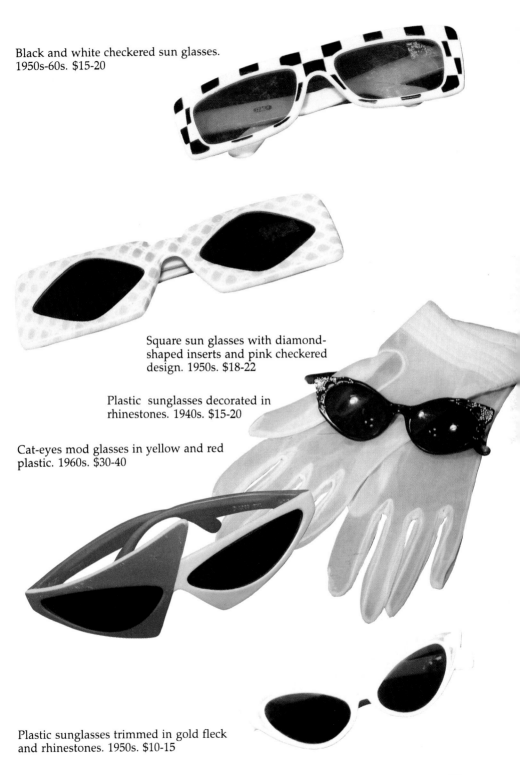

Black and white checkered sun glasses.
1950s-60s. $15-20

Square sun glasses with diamond-shaped inserts and pink checkered design. 1950s. $18-22

Plastic sunglasses decorated in rhinestones. 1940s. $15-20

Cat-eyes mod glasses in yellow and red plastic. 1960s. $30-40

Plastic sunglasses trimmed in gold fleck and rhinestones. 1950s. $10-15

Men's Clothing

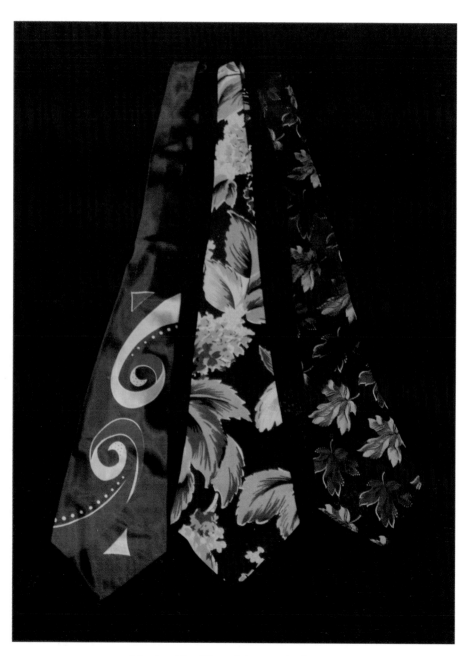

Men's wide silk neckties. 1950s. $15-20

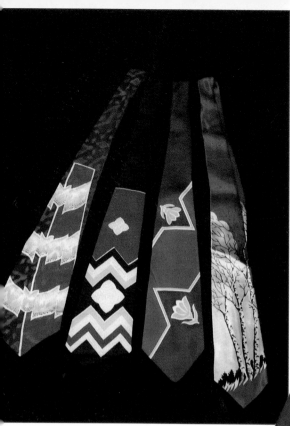

Wide silk design neck ties. 1940s. $10-14 each

Men's wide woven wool ties. 1950s. $10-15

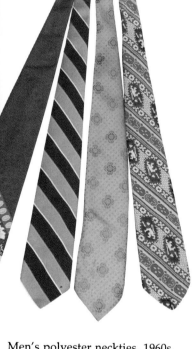

Men's polyester neckties. 1960s. $8-12

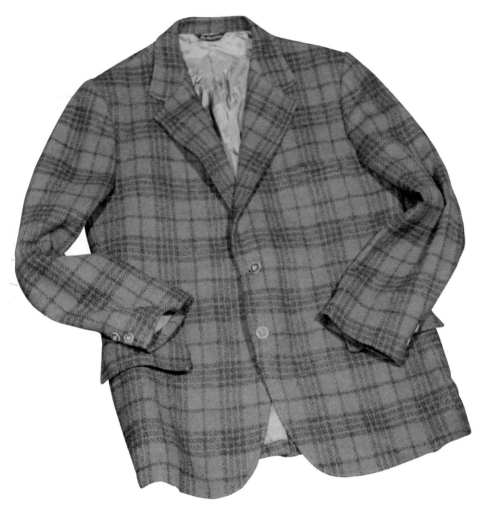

Man's wool checkered suit jacket. 1940s. $15-20

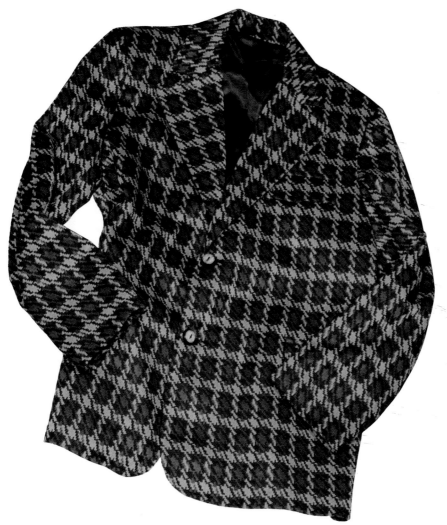

Man's double knit suit jacket. 1950s. $15-20

Jewelry

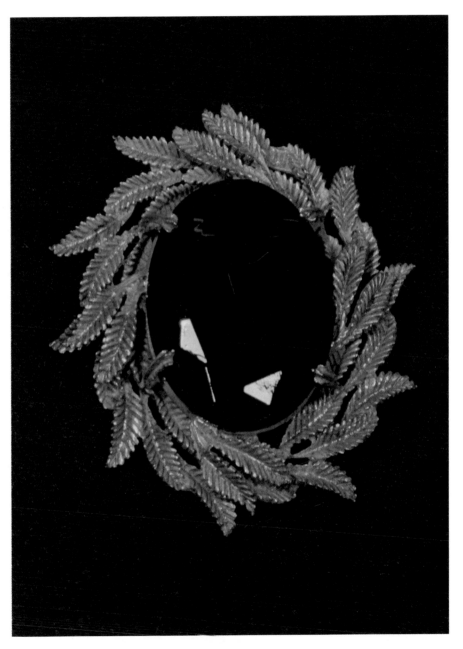

Gold tone broach with large amber center stone. 1950s. $20-30

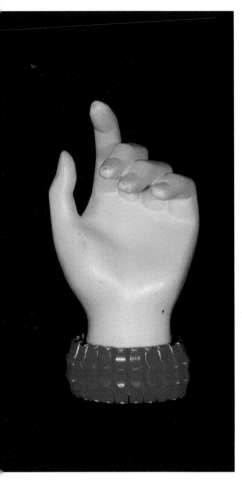 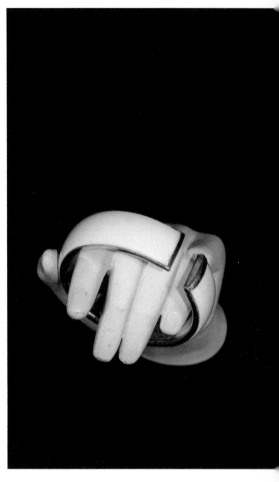

Plastic expandable bracelet. 1950s.
$15-20

Expandable bracelet. 1960s. $10-15

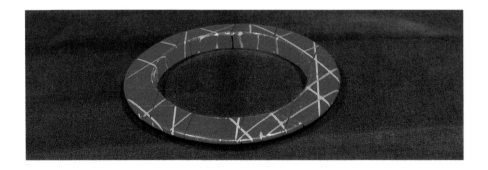

Wide plastic bracelet with string design. 1960s. $15-20

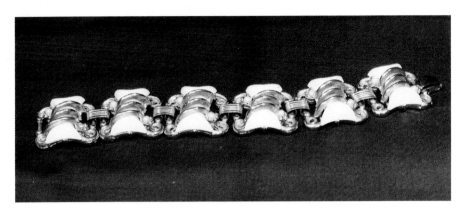

Gold-tone bracelet with bone-look plastic inserts. 1950s. $20-30

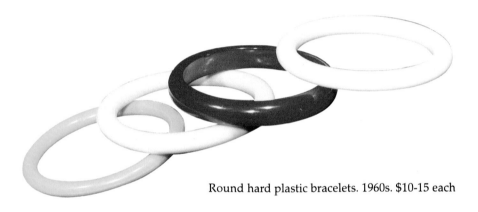

Round hard plastic bracelets. 1960s. $10-15 each

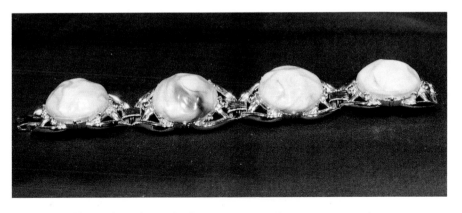

Gold-tone bracelet with plastic turquoise-like stones. 1950s. $25-35

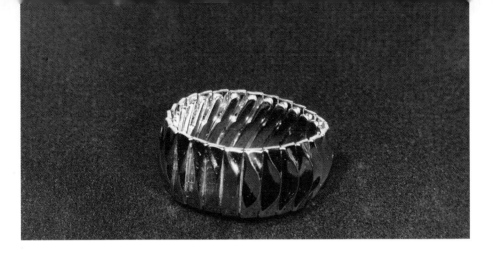

Silver stretch bracelet. 1950s. $15-20

Bracelet with hard plastic red and white
domino size squares on expandable
elastic. 1950s-60s. $30-40

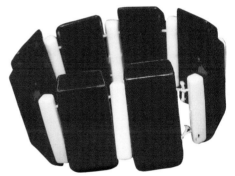

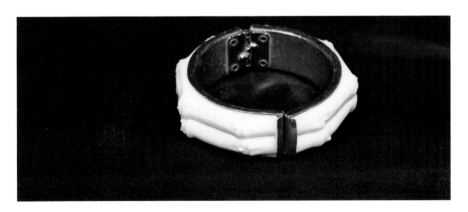

Gold-tone bracelet with bone-shaped inlaid plastic. 1950s-60s. $15-20

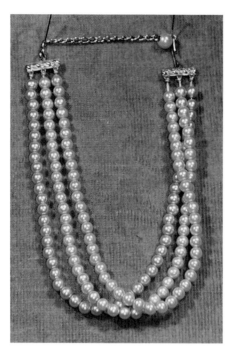

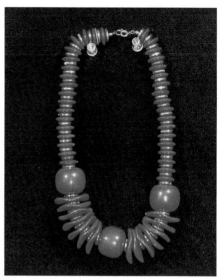

Red and gold plastic beads with large wavy disc spacers. "Hong Kong," 1960s. $15-20

Three-strand plastic pearl necklace. 1950s. $15- 22

Solid pink and swirl plastic beaded double necklace with gold spacers. 1960s. $10-15

Plastic yellow child's beads with single drop. 1950s. $20-30

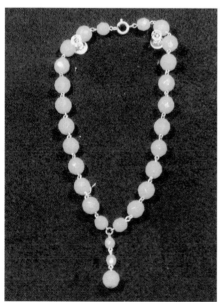

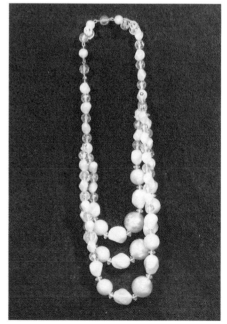

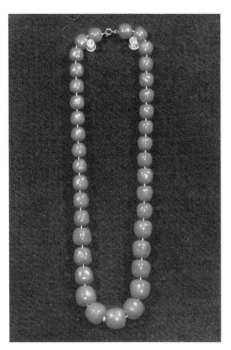

Salmon colored plastic beads with gold tone clasp. 1960s. $10-15

Frosted plastic swirl beads and clear plastic beads on this necklace with unusual matching clasps. 1940s. $15-20

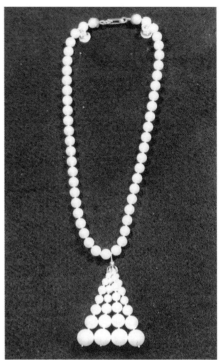

Light pink plastic single strand necklace with four strand tear drops. 1950s. $15-20

Faceted plastic red triple strand necklace. 1950s. $15-20

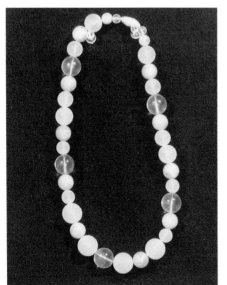

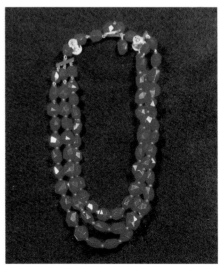

Multi-colored plastic beads with disc shaped spacers. Sterling clasp. 1960s. $15-20

Plastic triple strands of beads with glass spacers. 1960s. $20-25

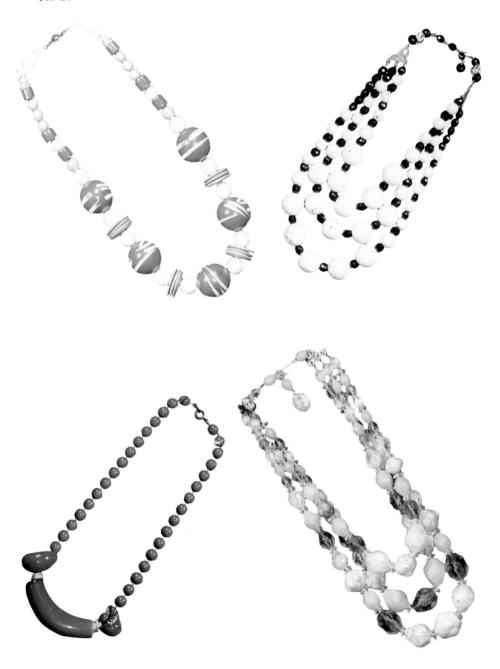

Jade green beads with brass spacers. Jade drop. 1940s. $30-40

Triple strands of cork beads with unusual faceted plastic spacers. 1940s. $20-25

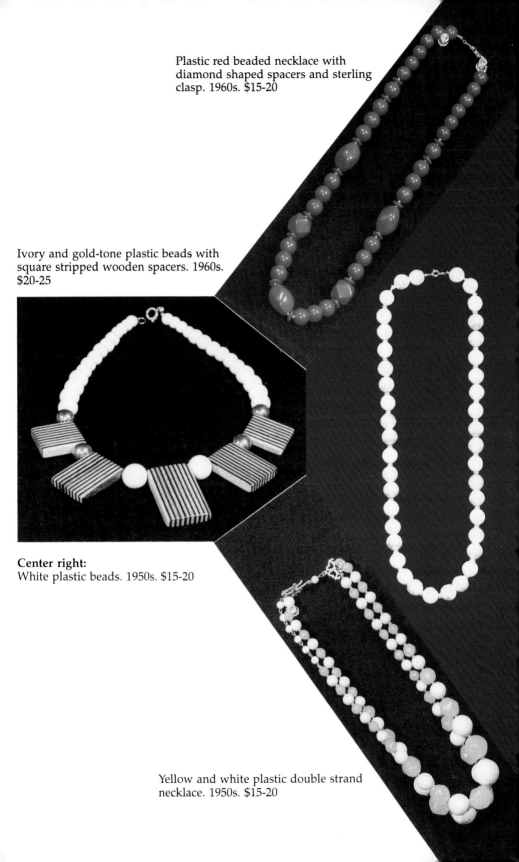

Plastic red beaded necklace with diamond shaped spacers and sterling clasp. 1960s. $15-20

Ivory and gold-tone plastic beads with square stripped wooden spacers. 1960s. $20-25

Center right:
White plastic beads. 1950s. $15-20

Yellow and white plastic double strand necklace. 1950s. $15-20

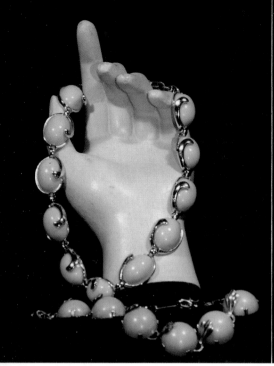

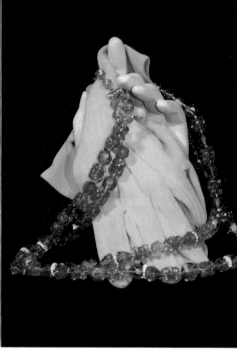

Two necklaces, one with blue round plastic beads and other with pink oval plastic beads in metal frames. 1950s. $14-20 each.

Amber colored bead necklace with silver spacers. "West Germany," 1950s. $20-30

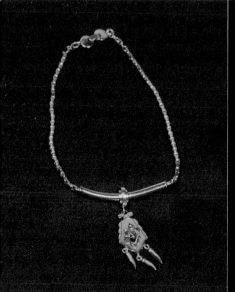

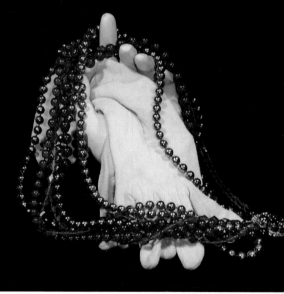

Chain necklace with designer drop and small stone inserted in center. 1960s. $30-40

Seven-strand necklace with multi-shaped blue plastic beads and beaded clasp. 1950s. $25-35

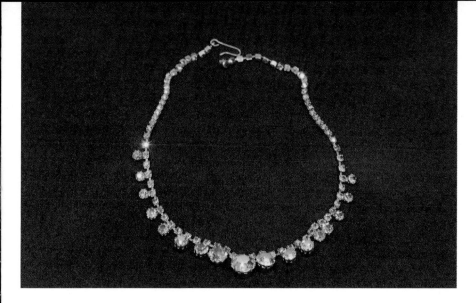

Rhinestone necklace. 1950s. $30-40

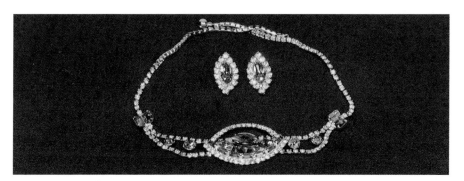

Rhinestone necklace and earrings. Smoke color. 1950s. $40-50

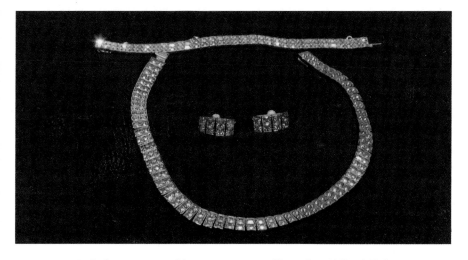

Pink rhinestone necklace, earrings, and bracelet. 1960s. $60-85

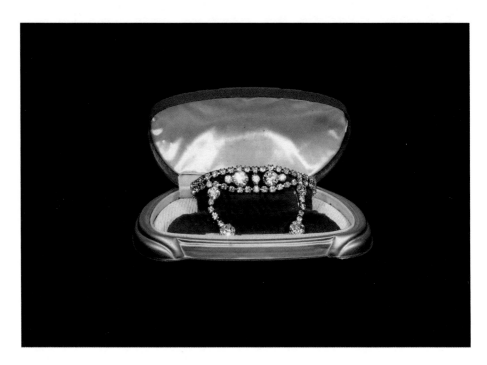

Rhinestone drop earrings and bracelet. 1950s. $40- 50

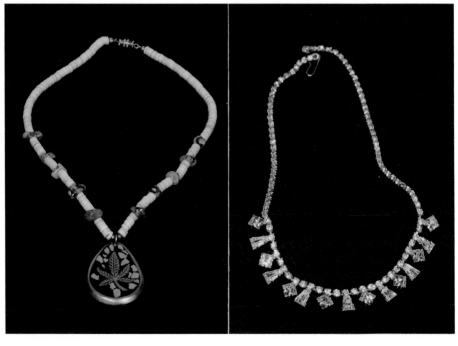

Turquoise necklace with marijuana leaf.
1960s. $30-40

Rhinestone necklace with replaced
clasp. 1950s. $30-40

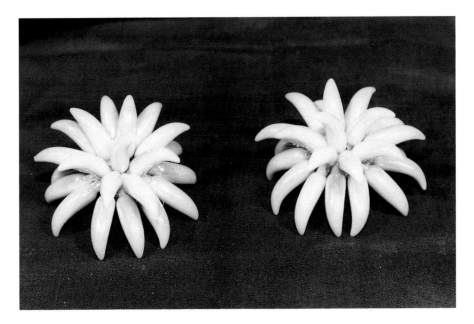

Flowers with banana-shaped petals make up these clip-on earrings. 1960s. $8-12

Gold-tone screw-on
earrings with
rhinestone centers.
1940s. $8-10

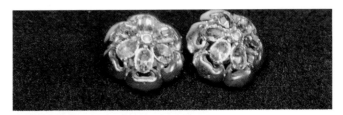

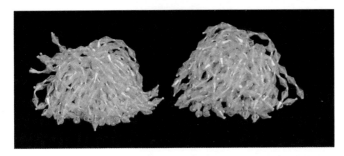

Plastic beaded shoe
clips. 1950s. $12-16

Shoe clips with
burlap base and
plastic vegetables.
1960s. $10-15

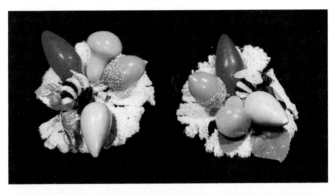

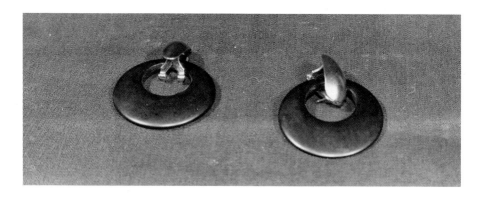

Plastic clip-on earrings. 1960s. $7-10

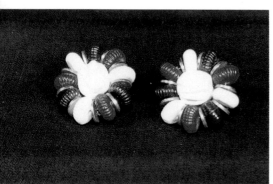

Red, white, and blue plastic discs with large pearl in center. 1960s. $8-12

Plastic discs and beads make up these clip-on earrings. 1960s. $6-10

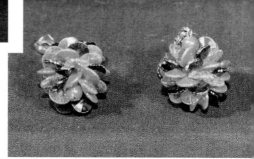

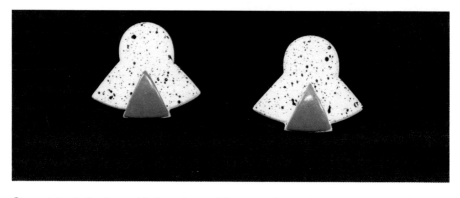

Geometric pin-back speckled earrings with green plastic ringer inserts. 1960s-70s. $6-10

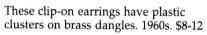

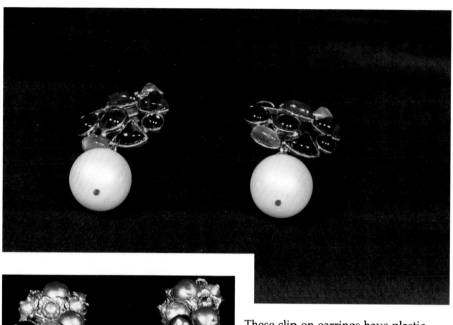

These clip-on earrings have plastic clusters on brass dangles. 1960s. $8-12

Long multi-colored grape cluster beads. Clip-on earrings. 1970s. $10-15

Metal frame with several different colored and shaped beads and a large pearl drop. 1960s. $10-15

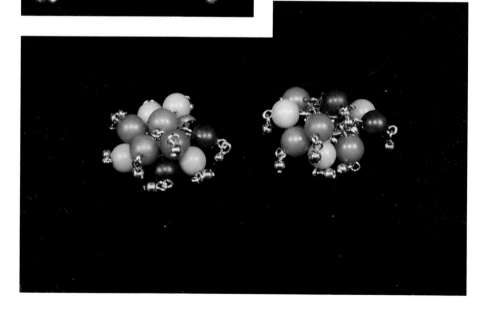

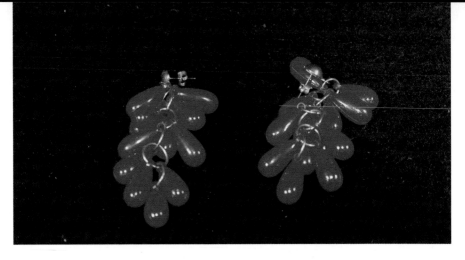

Red plastic dangle cluster pierced earrings. 1960s. $12-18

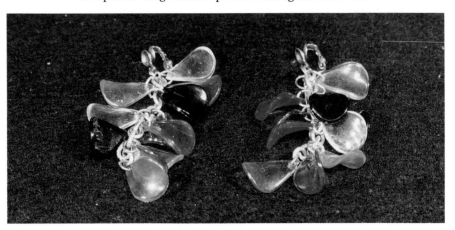

Multi-colored petal cluster plastic earrings, on silver chain. Pierced. 1960s. $10-15

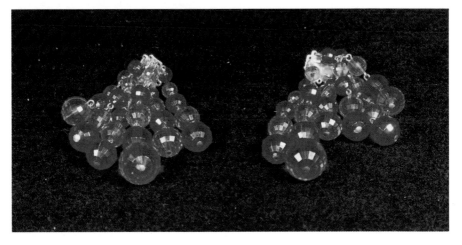

"Bobley" clip-on earrings with two-toned, faceted plastic bead clusters. 1950s-60s. $8-12

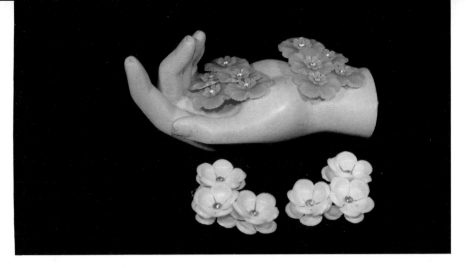

Clip-on earrings, with plastic flowers and rhinestones. 1950s-60s. $8-12

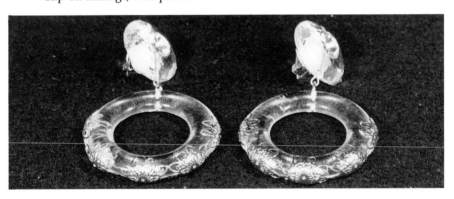

Large plastic bangles drop from these clip-on earrings with rhinestone centers. 1960s. $12-15

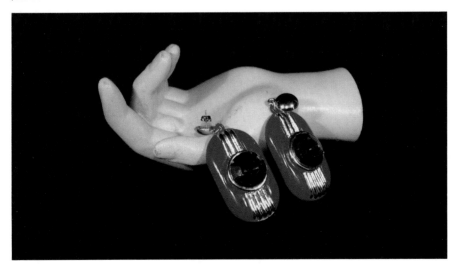

Red plastic oval clip-on earrings with gold wash and rhinestone inserts. 1960s. $10-15

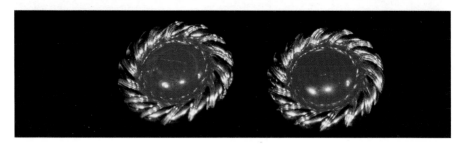

Clip-on earrings with gold-tone rope around large red centers. "Made in Italy," 1960s. $8-12

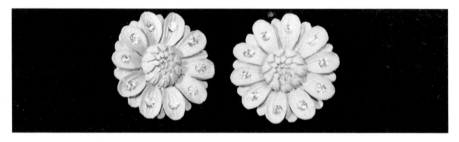

Floral clip-on earrings with rhinestones. 1950s-60s. $8-12

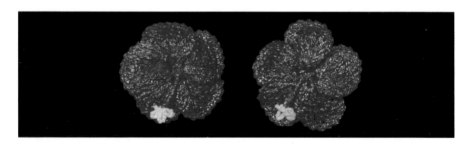

Earrings, red crochet-look flowers with plastic coating and yellow accents. 1960s. $10-15

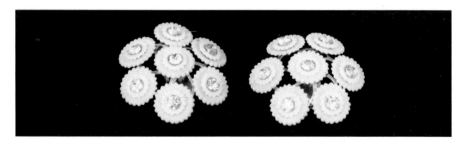

Plastic flowers with rhinestone inserts decorate these clip-on earrings. 1950s-60s. $8-12

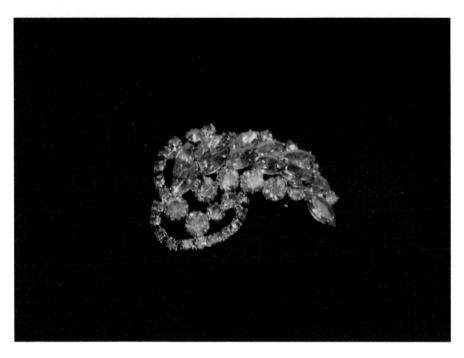

Green rhinestone broach. 1950s. $30- 40

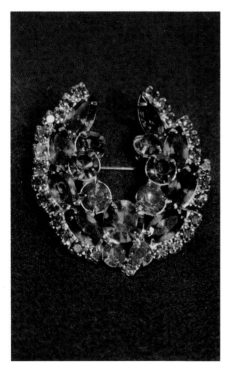

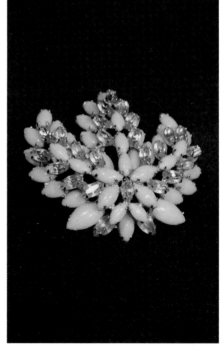

Rhinestone blue and green broach.
1950s. $30-40

Pink and white rhinestone broach.
1940s-50s. $30-40

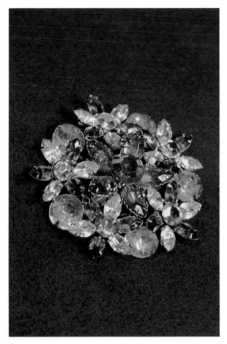

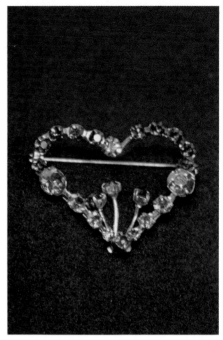

Two-tone green rhinestone broach.
1950s. $35-45

Heart-shaped rhinestone pin. "Coro."
1950s. $20-30

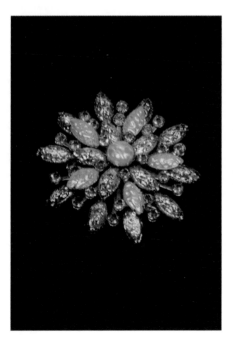

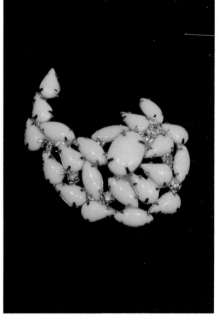

Rhinestone and pearl glitter broach.
1950s. $20-30

White stone and rhinestone broach.
1940s-50s. $20-30

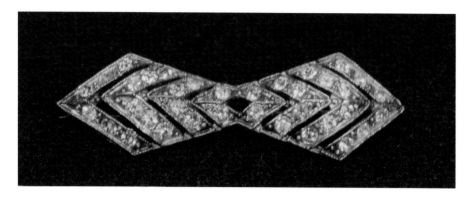

Rhinestone bow-shaped pin. 1940s. $20-30

Gold-tone flower pin with rhinestone center and green stones leaves. 1960s. $20-30

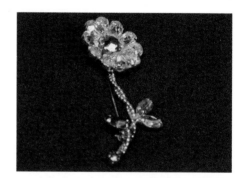

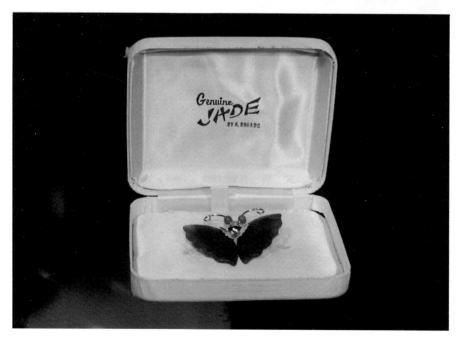

Jade butterfly pin. 1940s. $40-50

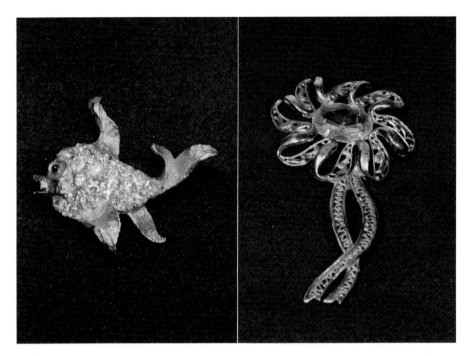

Gold-tone fish pin with rhinestone
decoration. 1960s. $20-30

Gold-tone flower pin with large gold
colored stone in center. 1960s. $20-30

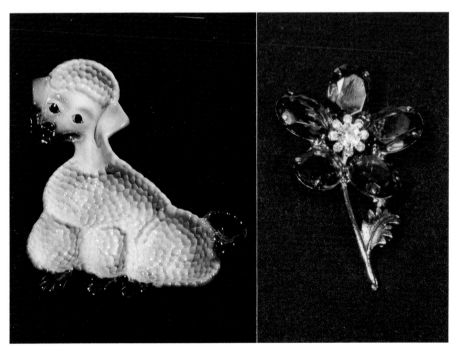

Pot metal poodle pin. 1960s. $15-20

Rhinestone flower pin. 1960s. $30-40

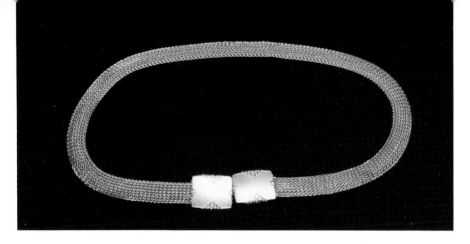

Metal woven belt with plastic pearlized buckle. 1940s. $15-20

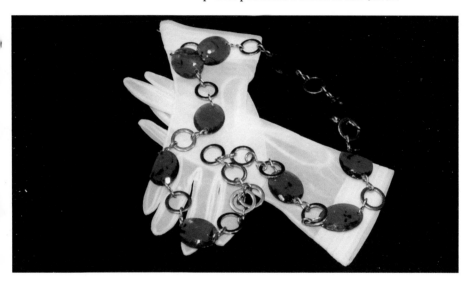

Tortoise shell circular beads and metal loop chain. 1950s. $15-20

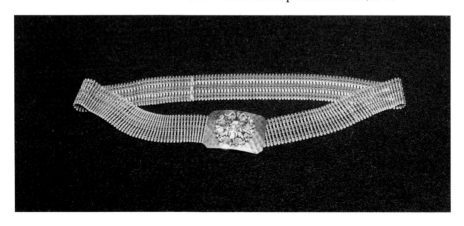

Metal weave chain belt with metal hook buckle. 1950s. $15-20

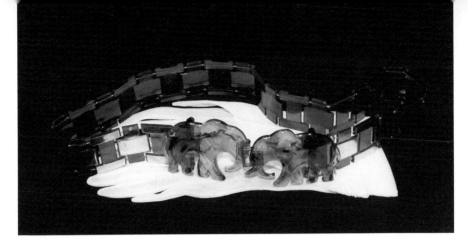

Tortoise shell and gold tone link belt with elephant connecting trunks for closure. 1950s. $20-30

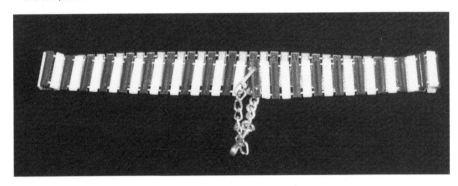

Plastic and metal belt with front drop chain. 1960s. $10-15.

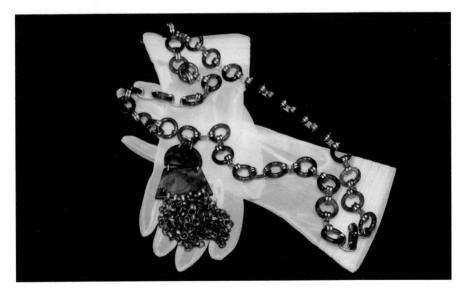

Tortoise shell ring chain belt with tortoise shell front drop with connected links. 1950s. $20-30

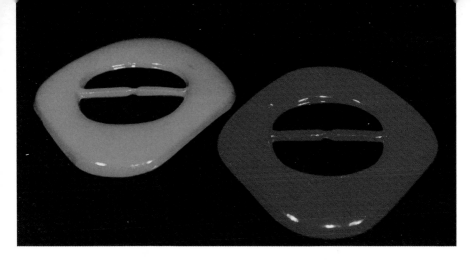

Plastic belt buckles. 1950s. $4-6 each

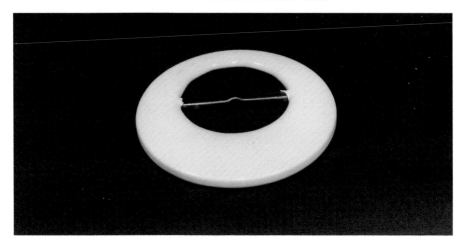

Plastic belt buckle. 1950s. $4-6

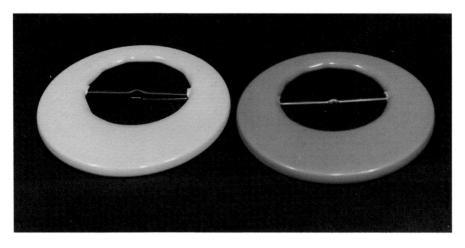

Orange and aqua plastic belt buckles. 1960s. $5-6 each

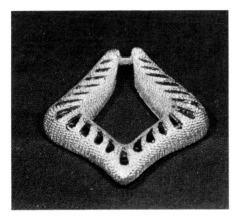

Pot metal belt buckle in gold-tone with plastic stones. 1960s. $5-8

Brass marijuana leaf belt buckle. 1960s. $25-35

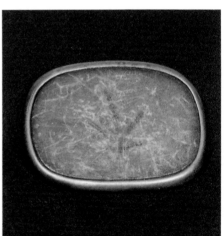

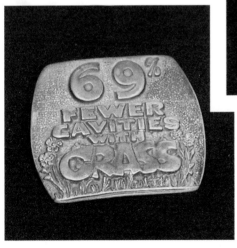

Brass belt buckle. 1960s. $20-30

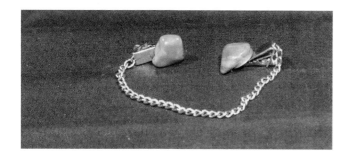

Chain sweater guard with plastic stone
trim on the ends. 1950s-60s. $15-20

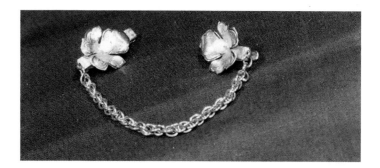

Gold-tone sweater guard with plastic
pearls set in the centers of the clips.
1950s-60s. $15-20

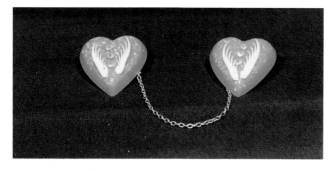

Metal chain with heart-shaped clips
embossed with feathers. 1950s-60s.
$15-20

Bibliography

Collector News & the Antique Reporter. Volume 35, number 11. March, 1995. Grundy Center, Iowa.

Collector News & The Antique Reporter. Volume 36, number 5. September, 1995. Grundy Center, Iowa.

Spiegel Catalog. The Golden Book. Spring & Summer. 1962. Chicago, Illinois.

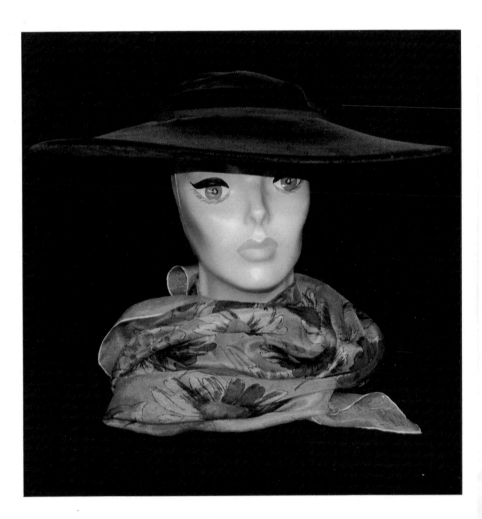